Everything You Need to Know About the New Wuhan 2020 Outbreak, Pandemic Spread and Symptoms

DR. ELLIOT G. CARSON

To Jack and Phoebe, my beloved patients..

INTRODUCTION

Don't panic, do prepare. With these four words, this hand novel begins the vital effort that will see you take power back from your fears and this disease.

As of the time of the writing of this novel, complete on the first day of February 2020, the 2019 Novel Coronavirus, (NCov19), which this novel will simply refer to as the Coronavirus, and any affiliated strains which emerge, is a still evolving public health threat whose full risk cannot yet be apprehended. What we know already is highly concerning, as massive quarantines have essentially seen millions of people in China, starting from the focal point of the outbreak in Wuhan, confined to their homes.

An information blackout imposed by the Communist Party of China under threat of incarceration has strangled the flow of videos, reports, and social media emerging from that country, even as we see mounting evidence that an incredibly dangerous pandemic has been released.

This is something we must prepare to face in our countries as initial indications suggest this virus has broken out of China and is presently infecting nations worldwide. Depending upon when you see this, the situation may be more or less advanced, so in preparation for what may happen, this volume will offer guidance for every step of the way about prudent precautions you must take to protect your family, what choices you will face in the challenging situation likely to emerge, and how to minimize risk to give yourselves the very best chance of survival and avoiding this health danger.

We will likely not know the full danger of this disease until

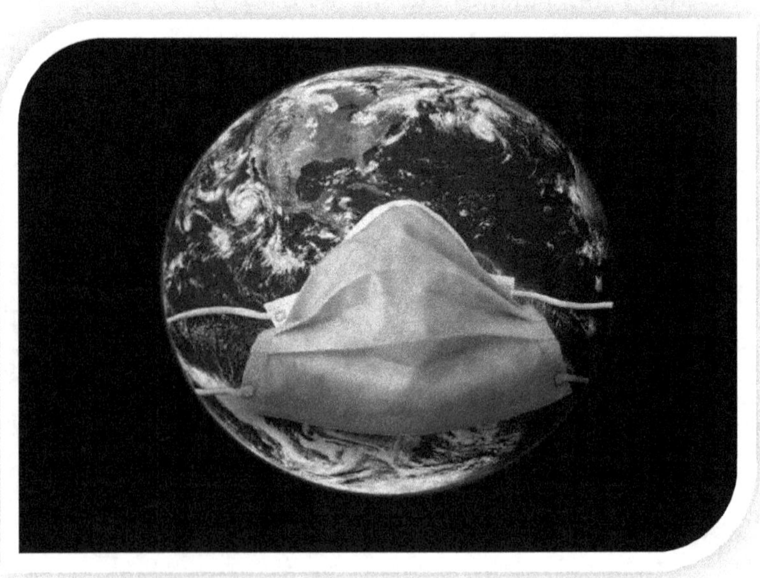

well after the threat has been established, so the first thing you must understand is that while Surviving Coronavirus will give you the tools you need to overcome most situations, it is impossible to predict all possible developments and to precisely chart the process by which the Coronavirus will evolve. As this virus has a high potential for mutation, what is true at the beginning of this outbreak may not remain true for the duration of events, so in recognition of that, this volume will teach you how to gather quality information from diverse sources. You will learn the basics of how viruses work, what key attributes determine the severity and transmissibility of a disease, and come to understand the most important fact which is if you wait until the virus is present, you've failed in the most basic preparation: To avoid trouble.

Depending upon who you believe, Coronavirus has an initial posted lethality rate between 2% and 11%, based upon mainstream medical sources who are using reported figures from the Chinese authorities to make their assessments. There are good reasons to doubt the veracity of these numbers in the direction as having substantially underestimated the risk which we will describe, but even these figures suggest a chance of death from the disease ranges from 1/40 to 1/10 or worse. If this becomes a global pandemic as it appears it will, that means a potential death toll upwards of nine figures, an event unseen in human history which would dwarf both the

Spanish Flu after World War I and the Black Plague of the late Middle Ages.

As terrible as this virus appears to be on its own, worse still might be the many disruptions this could cause to the normal functioning of our society. As public awareness about the severity of the Coronavirus rises, what will happen is panic leading to social unrest, increased criminality, rapid depletion of resources, and absenteeism. In concert with the spreading of this disease, expect to also see the inability of the medical system to provide adequate care to those who have the virus or who have other needs that require constant attention. As this break and as you will want and need greater access to medical professionals, it is likely they will be incredibly difficult to access beyond the first days of any major event that might precipitate. Furthermore, since this is already flu season and there are significant overlaps between the symptoms of coughing and infected lungs, it is highly probable that going to any medical facility either as a healthy person or with an ordinary sickness massively will increase your risk of exposure to the Coronavirus forcing you to decide if that chance is worth the benefit of medical advice.

While there is little doubt the government and international organizations such as the Centers for Disease Control (CDC) and World Health Organization (WHO) will be mobilizing all their resources toward combatting this outbreak, their understanding of the secondary risks of economic and social breakdown, which political forces will impose upon them, will lead them to continuously and deliberately present the most conservative estimations about the impact of this disease. Such caution might be warranted on their part, but this volume presumes the opposite in its orientation, that sound preparation consists of preparing for the worst-case scenario. You will never regret over preparing for something that does not happen more than you will regret not being ready for something truly terrible which does occur.

It would be impossible to predict every risk which will emerge during this difficult time, but the key to preparation is to make sure that instead of trying to understand these dangers perfectly and react to them, let us instead adopt a proactive mindset which takes power back for you and your loved ones. We definitely can assess our basic needs; can anticipate what logical precautions and preparation we need to take for health, safety, and survival. The sooner we act, the better our chances will be, but even for those with very limited means acting proximate than would be ideal, there are still options available to you which may prove of assistance.

As stressful as this situation might be, it is important to keep as clear a mind as possible, to use reason to patiently and continuously be mindful of new developments, and to act deliberately for your own safety. The best tool we all have during any dangerous situation is the fullest use of all our faculties and the hope is this guide will serve to allow you to ask the right questions and find the answers you need.

To get you started, much effort will be dedicated to the basic goods you should procure at the earliest opportunity to survive. For around 100 dollars, most of those items most essential to survival can still be gathered. From there, options are presented which will augment and bolster your ability to thrive, with the requirement that you figure out what needs are most crucial for your specific situation and family needs.

Lastly, a branch is included about what you might do should you believe you have contracted the Coronavirus. But as this threat is real, we will address it presenting a levelheaded view of your options, how you can bolster your body in its fight, allowing you to make an informed choice about whether you seek medical care.

The single goal of this volume is to empower you to survive and overcome the Coronavirus or any other pandemic threat. Writing with the decades of experience in personal preparation as a lifestyle, you should know as you take control of what you can, you will feel greater confidence as you assume greater security. We are hardwired to survive, and you are too!

As of February 26, 2020, the number of COVID-19 coronavirus-related cases reported stood at 81,260 across over 45 countries, which shows you just how fast the virus is spreading. On the other hand, the death toll is at 2,770 with 2,715 of those coming from China. Japan, France, Philippines, and Hong Kong have all recorded one death each. Iran has suffered 19 deaths, while Italy and Republic of Korea had 12 deaths.

In January 2020, The World Health Organization declared corona COVID-19 a global health emergency, which makes it the 6th disease ever to have that designation. Since then, the virus has been making headlines across the globe. The virus has now become the subject of thousands, if not millions proximate conversations.

Coronavirus is all over the TV, internet and newspapers - but what is it exactly? How is it transmitted? What does it do to you? Should you be worried? Is there a cure or vaccine?

I thought it would be very useful for myself and my family and others around the world to have a simple book detailing what we know so far about Coronavirus Covid-19 - so I have assembled reliable information from the WHO and CDC as well as other international resources to detail on what is

Corona Virus it is, how it spreads, who is most at risk and the answers to a whole plethora of questions.

WUHAN: THE CITY BEFORE THE OUTBREAK

On the 30th of December, 2019, he suggested that the utmost care and protocol be established as he suspected an impending outbreak after seeing the symptoms in seven patients. Little did Dr. Li Wenliang know at the time that he himself had already contracted the virus from one of his patients? Dr. Li would proximate succumb to his illness, at which time the outbreak would have been declared a global emergency by the World Health Organization.

The outbreak of 2019/2020 is caused by Wuhan, the capital of Hubei province, China, is believed to the ground zero of the outbreak. This became a cause for concern when over 41 people presented with symptoms of pneumonia with no apparent cause. Usually, it would take about 2 to 14 days of being exposed before symptoms begin to show in a person and at about this time before the symptoms are obvious, a person can still infect another, usually by aerosol and cough droplets.

The common symptoms reported are as follows:

- **Fever**

- **Cough**
- **Shortness of breath**
- **Pain in the muscles**
- **Tiredness**

Afterwards, the infected person may present with more severe symptoms such as respiratory distress and pneumonia which may eventually lead to death.

Currently, there are no known vaccines for the virus and currently available antiviral drugs are being tested for their ability to treat the condition.

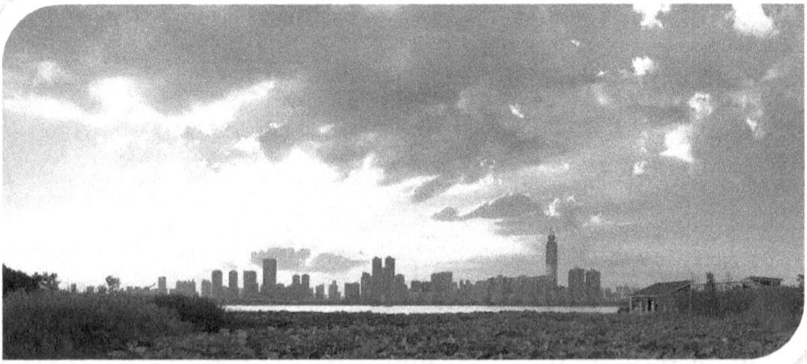

There is currently over 70,000 reported cases and 11,298 of them are in serious conditions. So far, 1,775 people have been killed by the virus. The rapid spread of the virus across mainland China and globally (with over 27 countries reporting at least one case each), can be explained by the strategic location of Wuhan in the Hubei province. As the seventh largest city in China and with a population of over 11 million people, it is a pivotal business and academic city with direct rail transportation interlinking all other major regions of China, as well as a major flight stop over from other international cities. Many unsuspecting commuters have been the conduit via which the virus has spread so fast, even before it was declared an outbreak. Wuhan's railway system is directly linked to Beijing to the south, Shanghai to the west as well as the North of Hong Kong.

The world health organization however, has further categorized the outbreak as a Public health emergency of international concern (PHEIC). With this label, China and indeed the world has set out to impose travel restrictions and quarantine measures. Airports and train stations across the world have instituted measures such as body temperature checks and health declarations among travelers as a means of raising the suspicion index and easing the identification of potentially infected persons. The virus is believed to have been contracted from animals, specifically bats. This assumption is however yet to be confirmed, though it has remained the working theory across the world owing to the earlier known information of other corona viruses having bats as their host, as well as the city of Wuhan housing a seafood market, Huanan Seafood Wholesale Market where exotic animals such as bats, pheasants, snakes, and deers are being sold for food. It is around this region that the outbreak was first reported.

Although corona viruses are known to also affect other animals, they have been established in earlier branch to evolve virulent strains that affect humans adversely, as was the case with SARS. Such variants as explained earlier, have the capacity to be transmitted from one human to another via respiratory droplets. Among the first seven documented cases, two were linked to the Sea Food market. Although Dr Li's outcry of a possible outbreak was on the 30th of December, a publication by Chinese epidemiologists on the 1st of January, 2020 shows that the first cluster patients who presented with pneumonia of unknown cause had been noted on the 21st of December, 2019. On the 21st of December, the Singaporean Ministry of health reported a case of pneumonia of an unknown cause as well.

By 31 December, 2019, China had issued a notice on the treatment of Pneumonia of unknown cause to the Wuhan municipal health center and this was followed immediately by a high scrutiny process in neighboring Taiwan, Hong Kong and Macau regions. And by January 1, the Huanan Seafood market was closed down by the Chinese government. But this measure proved to be too late as 41 people would present with the symptoms of the condition the following day, 27 of whom were directly exposed to the Huanan food market. On the 3rd of January, Chinese scientists had isolated three strains of the virus from samples collected from infected patients. However, this information was not made public to the world health organization until the January 9, 2020, at which time the world health organization then confirmed that the novel corona virus had been isolated from one person who had been hospitalized. The European center for disease prevention and control also on the same day posted a risk assessment protocol. In ground zero China, the CCTV reported that a new corona virus had been found in 15 of 57 patients with the illness in the city of Wuhan.

Fudan University had posted it on virological.org from Shanghai. Three other sequences were posted from the Chinese center for disease control and prevention, one other from the Chinese academy of medical sciences another from Jinyintan hospital in Wuhan. All sequences where uploaded to the Global Initiative on Sharing All Influenza Data (GISAID) portal.

January 11, the World health organization published its initial guidelines on travel advice, testing in the laboratory and medical investigation. While in China, 700 contacts of the

41 confirmed cases had been located and monitored for signs.

January 13, Thailand witnessed her first confirmed case of novel corona virus, the first confirmed case outside of China, a 61-year-old woman whose residence is in Wuhan, China. She had arrived Bangkok on the 8th of January. Also, the United States CDC announced that the genome had been posted on National Institutes of Health (NIH) genetic sequence database, GENBANK.

January 15, the second death occurs, 69-year-old Chinese man succumbs to the disease. A diagnostic protocol, developed by a team from Charitè Hospital was posted by the WHO.

January 16, a 30-year-old Chinese tested positive to the virus in Japan, as reported by the ministry of health, labour and welfare during his hospital stay.

January 17, Thailand confirms her second case while the confirmed cases in China rose to 45.

January 18, the city of Wuhan holds her annual banquet to mark the Chinese New Year. In attendance were forty thousand families, sharing food and utensils. It is possible that some people exposed to the virus may have been present on the said event and may have infected others. The mayor of

Wuhan would proximate state that the banquet had gone on because at the time, it was not known that the virus could be transmitted from one human to another.

January 19, just one day after the banquet, Wuhan reported an additional 136 laboratory confirmed cases, two others were confirmed in Beijing while another was also confirmed in Guangdong. One of the earlier confirmed cases in Wuhan died on this day, bringing the death toll to three in China.

Five people who attended a private international sales company meeting in Singapore with an attendance of 109 people, were confirmed to be infected with the virus. One of the attendees of this conference was from Wuhan, China. A buffet was said to have been held in the honor of the guests. This incident confirmed that the virus could actually spread from human to human, thereby raising the threat level according to the WHO.

January 21, cases across China's major cities including Shanghai and Beijing hit 291. At this time however, the center for global infectious disease analysis at imperial college London suggested the actual figure of infected persons to be 1700 while the university of Hongkong placed the figure at 1300 people. The confirmed deaths had gotten to 6 persons. Although Chinese officials had delayed themselves in the public reporting of the spread of the virus and had further under-reported the number of cases at a certain point and were not forthcoming with timely information to further prevent the spread of the virus.

January 22, new cases were reported in Macau and Hongkong and on the evening on this same day, a second was also reported from Hongkong. Furthermore, five other cases were also confirmed in Beijing and nine from Guangdong . Five more patients from Shangai and two from Tianjin , Zheijang five and Jiangxi one confirmed case. The total reported cases in China increased to 571 and the death toll to 17.

On the international scene, two new cases were reported in Thailand making Thailand cases a total of four. Officials in Wuhan announce a quarantine of greater Wuhan which was to commence the following day.

January 23, WHO Situation report: Jiangsu reported its first laboratory confirmed case. Heilongjiang reported its first two laboratory confirmed cases. Both Fujian and Guangxi reported an additional three laboratory confirmed cases. Xinjiang reported two laboratory confirmed cases. Shaanxi reported three laboratory confirmed cases. Gansu reported two confirmed cases. Macau also reported its second laboratory confirmed case, another 66-year old man from

Wuhan. In all the total number of laboratories confirmed cases in mainland China increased to 628 while the death toll remained at 17.

Singapore reported its first laboratory confirmed case, a 66-year-old man from China. Vietnam confirmed its first two laboratory confirmed case, a 65-year-old father and a 27 year old son from China.

January 24, WHO Situation Report 4: Shandong reported six additional laboratory confirmed cases. Huanan reported 15 additional laboratory confirmed cases. Liaoning reported one additional laboratory confirmed case. Fujian reported four additional laboratory confirmed cases. Anhui reported six additional laboratory confirmed cases. Ningxia reported one additional laboratory confirmed case. Shanghai reported 13 more laboratory confirmed cases, bringing the total to 33 new cases.

Japan, South Korea and the United States reported their second cases.

The first confirmed incidence of human to human transmission outside of China was documented by WHO in Vietnam.

January 25, WHO Situation Report 5: Australia confirmed its first four cases, one in Victoria and three in New South

Wales. Japan conformed its third case.

January 26, WHO Situation Report 6:

Two of which are from California and one in Arizona. Hongkong confirmed its sixth to eight cases. Thailand confirmed its eight case. 39 suspected cases were awaiting laboratory confirmation.

The Chinese center for disease control and prevention started working on vaccines for the virus. Health officials in Ivory Coast announced a suspected case of corona virus infection. WHO director general, Tedros Ghebreyesus traveled to Beijing to confer with Chinese officials and health experts on corona virus.

China started requiring nationwide use of monitoring stations for screening, identification and immediate isolation of Coronavirus-infected travelers, including at airports, railways stations, bus stations and ports.

A tentative clinical profile of the new corona virus was published by an assistant professor of population health science at the Icahn school of medicine at Mount Sinai in New York. The Lethality of the virus is unknown; however, the death toll had claimed to above three percent.

Wiang Xianliang, a Hubei provincial government official, died of pneumonia caused by the virus.

Cambodia confirmed its first case of the virus, a Chinese man who came with his family to Sihanneukville Singapore confirmed a fifth case, a 56-year-old Chinese national who arrived from Wuhan on 18 January. Germany confirmed its first case in Bavaria, a case of domestic transmission.

Taiwan reports its first case of domestic transmission of the coronavirus.

Beijing reports first death from coronavirus.

In Germany, the first specific, global case of coronavirus being transmitted by a person with no symptoms has been reported. The originally-infected individual is from Shanghai.

January 28, WHO situation reports 8: bringing the total infected there to 14. Singapore confirms two more cases, bringing the total infected in Singapore to seven. That was followed by a Hubei-related suspension from 29 January.

Germany confirmed 3 new cases, all of whom were co-workers of the first confirmed patient. France confirmed its fourth case, an elderly Chinese tourist who is in critical condition.

Scientists from The Peter Doherty Institute for Infection and Immunity (Doherty Institute) in Melbourne reported that they had successfully grown 2019-nCoV from a patient sample.

Companies in Hubei are required not to resume services before 13 February, and schools in Hubei are to postpone the reopening of schools.

Outbreaks of coronavirus- related diseases

Outbreaks of coronavirus types of relatively high mortality are as follows:

OUTBREAKS	VIRUS TYPE	DEATH TOLL
2003 severe acute respirat outbreaks	SARS-CoV	774
2012 middle East respirato syndrome	MERS-	Over 400
2018 middle East respiratory syndrome	MERS-	41
2019-20 coronavirus outbreaks	SARS- Cov 2	Over 2600

WHAT IS A PANDEMIC

On February 2, 2020, The New York Times quoted the director of the U.S. National Institute of Allergy and Infectious Diseases as saying that the Wuhan coronavirus was poised to "almost certainly" become a pandemic.

The word 'pandemic' has ominous connotations for most

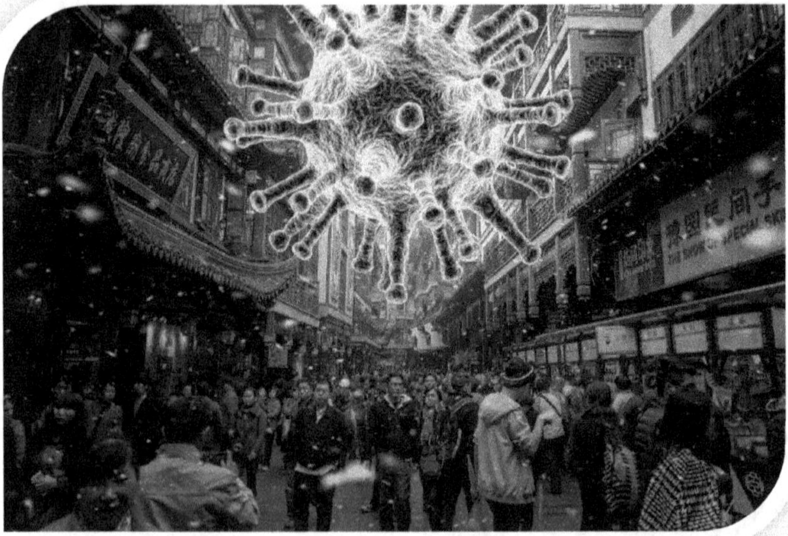

people. This isn't without just cause, but it's important to ensure that you're able to put the term into proper perspective.

A pandemic is an epidemic outbreak that occurs on at least two continents at the same time. So, what's an epidemic? To get this designation, a community (which can mean a city, state, country, or a continent) needs to experience a sudden and unexpected increase in the number of cases confirmed of one specific illness.

Some people (and even historical resources) use the terms epidemic and pandemic interchangeably. Technically, though, an epidemic doesn't take place in more than one continent at once.

Examples of Epidemics

- *2015 Indian Swine Flu Outbreak (2,035 deaths)*
- *2013-2016 West Africa Ebola Virus Epidemic (approximately 11,300 deaths)*
- *1910-1912 Bubonic Plague Outbreak in China (40,000 deaths)*
- *1772 Plague Outbreak in Persia (approximately 2 million deaths)*

- *1707-1709 Iceland's Great Smallpox Epidemic (18,000 deaths, 36 percent of the country's population)*

Examples of Pandemics

- *1331-1353 Black Death Plague in Europe, Asia, and North Africa (between 75-200 million estimated deaths, 30-60 percent of the population)*

- *1889-1890 Worldwide Flu Pandemic (1 million deaths)*

- *1918-1920 Worldwide Spanish Flu (estimated up to 100 million deaths)*

- *1960-present Worldwide HIV/AIDS Pandemic (approximately 30 million deaths)*

- *2009 Worldwide Flu Pandemic (203,000 deaths)*

What is the difference of Endemic vs Epidemic vs Pandemic?

Often there is confusion between the meaning of Endemic, Epidemic and Pandemic. Here what they mean.

Endemic, a disease that affects permanently the population of a particular region of the world. For example, Malaria constitute an ongoing worry in parts of Africa. It occurs at a predictable rate in some area or among a set population.

Epidemic Since 2010 14 epidemics since 2010 have been recorded.

Is the COVID-19 a Pandemic? As from what stated by the WHO in, COVID-19 it is not at the level of a Pandemic.

WHAT IS CORONAVIRUS

Coronaviruses are a group of viruses that cause diseases from the common cold to more serious diseases like SARS and Middle East Respiratory Syndrome (MERS), according to the World Health Organization (WHO).

Originally, these viruses were spread among animals and humans. SARS, for example, was thought to have been spread to people from civet cats when MERS transferred to humans from the camel type. Among species that have not yet bitten humans, many known coronaviruses circulate.

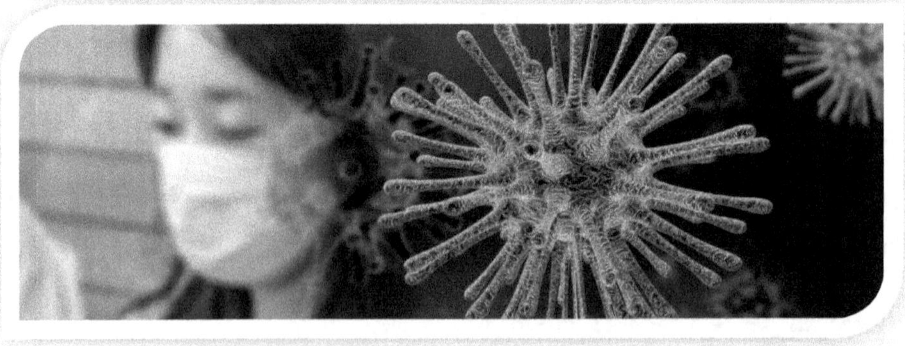

The name Coronavirus is derived from the Latin word

crown or halo. The picture of the virus is reminiscent of a solar corona under an electron microscope. A novel coronavirus found on 7 January 2020 and named 2019-nCoV by the Chinese authorities is a new strain not earlier identified in humans.

It is little understood, even though transmission from human to human has been confirmed.

The coronavirus incubation period remains unknown. Some sources say that it could take 10 to 14 days.

The number one question you must be asking yourselves right now is, "what is a coronavirus?"

Contrary to popular opinion, coronavirus is not a single virus, but a large family of viruses that infect birds, mammals, and humans. The coronaviruses cause illnesses ranging from the common cold to severe and devastating epidemics like Severe Acute Respiratory Syndrome (SARS-CoV), Middle East Respiratory Syndrome (MERS-CoV), and the now identified novel coronavirus (nCoV).

Corona virus, like every other virus, survives and thrives by a unique complex routine. Viruses in general are so small they cannot support a complete cell structure of their own and as a result, they cannot reproduce by themselves even by the basic biological definitions of reproduction; self-replication or division. To make up for this, they instead find a host cell in which they introduce their genetic materials. Using this as a template, just like a photocopying machine, the host cells then churns out new copies of the virus. So far, about five thousand viruses have been identified and classified. And in all, either RNA or DNA viruses, regardless of shape, their basic structures are usually the same. All viruses are made of a genetic material (DNA or RNA), a molecule which carries this genetic material and a protein coating which holds all these together. Some however may even have a fat envelope around them on which there are receptors that select which particular cells the virus will be attached to.

The journey into the discovery of viruses began 1884 when French scientist Charles Chamberlain came up with the idea of a filter with pores so small, even bacteria could not filter through them. It would be proximate known as the Chamberlain filter. This filter came in handy in Dmitri Ivanovsky's research in what was proximate identified to be the Tobacco mosaic virus, as the extracts gotten from the plant and filtered were shown to be still infective. But it wasn't until 1931 when the electron microscope was invented by German engineers Ernest Ruska and Max Knoll that a detailed image of a virus would be seen. After that, the earliest challenge in the study of viruses was how to grow them outside living animals. That breakthrough came in 1931 when the influenza virus was cultured in fertilized eggs, and then polio virus in cultures of living cells in 1949.

For viruses, their cycle comprises finding a host, attaching itself to that host, penetrating the cell wall, uncoating to release its genetic material and finally replicating. All these are evolutionary adaptive mechanisms for survival. But on the other side of the table is the effect this process has in the host animal. Usually, but not always, this process leads to a disease condition in the organism, depending on the part of the organism the virus has an affinity for and the virulence of the virus itself.

Corona virus gets its name from the same Latin word "Corona" which means "crown". This is so because of the fringes on the surface of the virus which is similar to that of a crown. They are single stranded RNA (Ribonucleic Acid) viruses with a genome size of about 26-32. It wasn't until the invention of the electron microscope that corona viruses were able be viewed and described in their details. The most common type of corona viruses found in the nasal cavity of people suffering from the common cold and another variant which causes infectious bronchitis in chickens were the first corona viruses to be identified. This common cold virus would come to be known as "human corona virus 229E and OC43". They belong to the order of Nidovirales and classified as a family called Coronaviridae. The spikes on the surface of the virus for which it earns its name is known as peplomers and this structure helps determine where the virus latches on to in its hosts. The virus is also made up of a membrane, an envelope and a nucleocapsid.

The oldest known common ancestor of the corona virus is about 10,000 years old according to consensus agreements, although they are believed to be much older than this. It is also known that bats and birds are the most common hosts for this virus. However, other more recent hosts like the civet cat, camels, and bovine groups of animals have become ideal hosts for the corona virus.

When a corona virus enters a host, the spike clings to a cell in the host while the virus makes its entry into the cell cytoplasm. While inside, the earliest process occurs, the virus sheds its coat thereby revealing the RNA genome within. This genome is what carries the details of the virus and with which other viruses can be made. The virus essentially turns the host cells into tiny manufacturing plants, using its own genetic details as a template for replication and churning out new viruses from the cell machinery.

The process is then repeated when a new host/human is infected, usually by respiratory droplets and aerosols from an infected person. In other cases, it is from the consumption of an infected animal as in the case of SARS and Covid-19.

Not all corona viruses can be passed from animals to humans. There are currently only seven know strains that affect humans:

- *Human Corona Virus 229E*
- *Human corona virus OC43*
- *Severe Acute Respiratory Syndrome Related Coronavirus (SARS-CoV)*
- *Human Corona Virus NL63*
- *Human corona virus HKU1*
- *Middle East Respiratory Syndrome Related Coronavirus (MERS-CoV)*
- *Novel Corona virus (COVID-19)*

Asides SARS, MERS and the Novel Corona virus, the other corona viruses listed above are implicated in the common cold and are constantly and continually being transmitted across the human population globally with no serious debilitating consequences.

CDC is sharply responding to the worldwide happening of

COVID-19 and making ready for the potential of community unfold within us.

What the scientific community and politics are doing right now

1. *Preparing initial responders, tending suppliers, and health systems*

2. *Establishing visibility across tending systems to grasp tending use significantly surges in demand for treatment and associated resources.*

3. *Conducting an in-depth research to clinical and hospital skilled organizations to confirm health system preparation.*

4. *Producing quite twenty-three steerage documents on infection management, hospital preparation assessments, and personal protecting instrumentation.*

5. *Working closely with tending facilities and suppliers to strengthen infection management principles that acknowledge PPE is one element of a bigger set of practices that facilitate to limit the unfold of sickness.*

6. *Developing a spread of respirator conservation methods, as well as methods to create provides last longer (such as victimization different merchandise like reusable respirators) and lengthening the*

utilization of disposable respirators is also thing to consider.

7. *Leverage existing telehealth tools to direct folks to the proper level of tending for his or her medical desires.*

8. *Working with provide chain partners to grasp provide usage, what merchandise are offered, and once additional aggressive measures may have to be taken to confirm that tending employees at highest risk have access to PPE.*

9. *Sharing data with stakeholders to assist them acknowledge once to shift the methods they're victimization.*

Ways government agency Protects and Prepares Communities

1. Reinforcing state, territorial, and native public health readiness

2. Coordinating with states to spot and mitigate gaps in readiness that may facilitate scale back the untold of sickness within the community whereas protective employees, infrastructure, and establishments.

3. Working with state and native public health to use existing Public Health Emergency preparation (PHEP) funding to support COVID-19 preparation and response activities is also what we need.

4. Leveraging funding mechanisms to assist states accelerate preparation activities.

5. Providing technical help and steerage to states to boost their ability to retort to the happening.

6. Supporting communities, businesses, and faculties

7. Creating business steerage to assist the general public and personal sectors guarantee they're able to operate with diversifications like telework and versatile leave of absence policies, still as the way to respond if associate worker gets sick.

8. Developing steerage for service programs, K-12 faculties, and colleges/universities to assist them set up and steel oneself against COVID-19 and respond if there's a neighborhood happening in their community.

9. Providers coming up with guides for COVID-19 that household, community- and faith-based organizations, event planners of mass gatherings, and public health communicators will use.

10. Educating communities regarding no pharmaceutical interventions (NPIs) that facilitate slow the untold of ill health, like COVID-19.

The Coronavirus (CoV) family has an inclination to evolve into deadly diseases and has regularly caused extreme sickness. Camels in the Middle East and maybe in East Africa keep on spreading the virus, which may require hospitalization, particularly in older people with the earlier co-morbidities.

In 2014, a solitary case caused a flare-up of 186 infections in South Korea while a proximate case from the Middle East was contained because of quick execution of general protective measures.

MERS-CoV continues to infect humans and, therefore, is recorded as a pathogen with pandemic potential by the World Health Organization (WHO) and the Coalition for Epidemic Preparedness Innovations (CEPI). Incidentally, there are no endorsed medications for MERS-CoV or some CoV.

In the daily newspapers and TV stations, people are panicking, and families are crying over the uncured coronavirus that has claimed the lives of so many. The country of origin has rushed to build several hospitals to accommodate the infected individuals. It is now a fact that researchers need the pathogen to investigate the rising disease rate and to create tests, medications, and immunizations. The Wall Street Journal, dated February 6, 2020, highlights the death rates of those who have contracted the virus. According to the news, China has isolated people infected with the virus, and many have to be quarantined.

What is this deadly virus that medical personnel are trying to fight and seek cures for? With no sign that an episode of another coronavirus is lessening, virologists worldwide are eager to get their hands-on physical examples of the infection. They are planning to test medications and antibodies, create models of the disease, and explore inquiries regarding the science of the infection, like how it spreads.

Also, according to the Wall Street Journal and other news outlets, little is known about this infection, which conveys the logical name 2019-nCoV, signifying "novel coronavirus." Scientists and health authorities are hastening to find out additional information. This new infection has a place with a group of infections known as coronaviruses, named for the crown-like spikes on their surfaces. They are spread for the most part by bats and pigs. The virus could transform effectively and can readily transfer from animals to people, starting with one human and then the nearest . As of late, they have become a developing player in unstoppable ailment flare-ups around the world.

These virus strains are known to cause diseases in the respiratory tract. Four of those strains cause basic colds. Concerns are about the perilous new infection behind a quick spreading pandemic in China. The quantity of individuals sick with or passing on viral pneumonia brought about by the new coronavirus is rising quickly, regardless of the isolation of a great many individuals and implementation of different measures in an attempt to stop it. The infection has been conveyed by tourists to different nations, including the United States of America.

Stress over the potential worldwide effect has disrupted international trade. The latest infection likely originated from bats. It isn't known precisely where or how it is transmitted to people, however. Health authorities said that the outbreak began in an enormous animal and fish wet market in Wuhan, China. Of the initial 41 cases, 27 were attendees at that market, as indicated by a report in The Lancet, a health magazine. However, three of the initial four individuals, who turned out to be sick on Dec. 1 and Dec. 10 said they had no contact with the market. An investigation by the New England Journal of Medicine found out that 55% of patients in Wuhan, who were already sick before Jan. 1, had a connection to the market compared to 8.6% of individuals who were infected after that point. Researchers stated that it will require some investigation to pinpoint the real source.

Human Coronaviruses (HCoVs) have for quite some time been viewed as insignificant pathogens, causing the "normal cold" in any individual. Nonetheless, in the 21st century, two profoundly pathogenic HCoVs—Severe Acute Respiratory Syndrome Coronavirus (SARS-CoV) and Middle East Respiratory Syndrome Coronavirus (MERS-CoV)— rose up from food supplies to cause worldwide pandemics with disturbing severity and mortality. A definitive degree and impact of this flare-up is uncertain at present as the situation is rapidly evolving.

Peri-domestic warm-blooded animals may fill in as middle hosts, encouraging recombination and changing with the development of hereditary variety. The surface spike (S) glycoprotein is a multifunctional molecular machine that mediates coronavirus entry into host cells.

Up to this point, HCoVs received generally little consideration. This changed in 2002 when instances of extreme atypical pneumonia were discovered in Guangdong Province, China, causing worry as the infection spread through international travel across two dozen countries. Palm civets and raccoon hounds were the first suspects; in any case, as more definitive information became accessible, agreement developed that bats were the characteristic hosts.

TAXONOMY

The scientific name for coronavirus is *Orthocoronavirinae* or *Coronaviridae.*

Genus: Alphacoronavirus.

Species: *Human coronavirus 229E, Human coronavirus NL63, Miniopterus bat coronavirus 1, Miniopterus bat coronavirus HKU8, Porcine epidemic diarrhea virus, Rhinolophus bat coronavirus HKU2, Scotophilus bat coronavirus 512*

Genus: Betacoronavirus.

Species: *Betacoronavirus 1, Human coronavirus HKU1, Murine coronavirus, Pipistrellus bat coronavirus HKU5, Rousettus bat coronavirus HKU9, Severe acute respiratory syndrome-related coronavirus, Tylonycteris bat coronavirus HKU4, Middle East respiratory syndrome-related coronavirus, Human coronavirus OC43, Hedgehog coronavirus 1 (EriCoV)*

Genus: Gamma Coronavirus.

Species: *Beluga whale coronavirus SW1, Infectious bronchitis virus*

Genus: Deltacoronavirus.

Species: *Bulbul coronavirus HKU11, Porcine coronavirus HKU15.*

A DEEP LOOK INTO CORONAVIRUS

According to Bhanu Sud, an infectious disease specialist, the word corona means '*crown*.' This disease got its name due to its crown-shaped appearance when viewed under an electron microscope.

Coronaviruses are majorly harmless, and they mostly cause mild to severe upper respiratory tract illnesses like the common cold. At some point in time, most people will get infected with these viruses.

For most people infected with these types of viruses, the outlook is usually good, while the MERS and SERS are to be dreaded.

10 percent of people with SARS usually die as a result of the virus, while 30% of the people living with MERS ends up with the same fate.

According to Bhayani, he has a feeling that this newly discovered virus has never been seen before. This is due to the fact that the virus is currently unknown, and the series of tests are continually being carried out to determine whether it has similarities with either MERS or SARS.

As earlier mentioned, coronaviruses mostly affect the respiratory tract of humans and other mammals. These viruses are often characterized by severe acute respiratory syndrome (SARS), cold, pneumonia, and the gut.

The first isolation of coronavirus was from an infectious bronchitis virus in birds. This has the ability to seriously devastate poultry stocks.

Around 15 to 30 percent of common colds are a resultant effect of these viruses.

In the last 70 years, scientists have discovered that cattle, dogs, pigs, horses, turkeys, cats, rats, and mice are all prone to coronaviruses infections. Of recent, China had a coronavirus outbreak that has extended into other countries.

The very first human coronaviruses (HCoV) were discovered in the 1960s. These viruses lived and survived in the noses of people with the common cold. OC43 and 229E are two coronaviruses that are infamous for a large proportion of common colds.

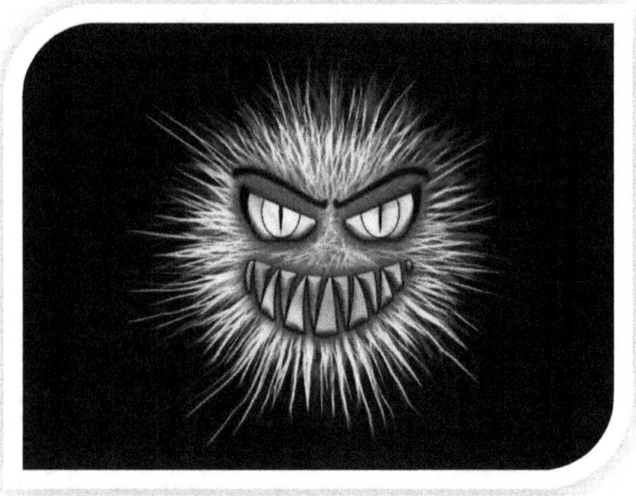

In Latin, "Corona" means "halo" or "crown." Scientists came about this name due to the crown-like projections on the surfaces of the viruses.

Coronavirus infections often occur in humans during winter and in early spring. It is a common occurrence for a person to become ill with a coronavirus induced cold, get better, then fall sick again a few months proximate due to the same reason.

This is so because the antibodies contained in coronavirus do not last for a very long time. The antibodies for a strain of coronavirus may also be useless against other strains.

What is Coronavirus and how did it originate?

Coronaviruses (CoV) are a big group of viruses that provoke illness. Illness can change from a common cold to more serious diseases. The most severe illness reportedly are:

- Severe Acute Respiratory Syndrome aka SARS-CoV (2003), originated in China

- Middle East Respiratory Syndrome aka MERS-CoV (2012), originated in Middle East

- Coronavirus (COVID-19 or nCoV) (2019), originated in China

Coronaviruses are defined as “zoonotic”, i.e. they are transmitted between animals and people.

There are a variety of other coronaviruses in animals that have not been passed to humans.

The infamous nCOV allegedly originated from an illegal wildlife market, which also doubles as a seafood market in Wuhan. A comparison of the new coronavirus and the old versions revealed that this new one originated from snakes.

According to Dr. Pooman Khetrapal Singh, who is the regional director of WHO South-East Region, the new coronavirus is being called coronavirus-2019. During the last meeting of the Emergency Committee of the International

Health Regulation, it was concluded that the outbreak of this virus is not declared as a public health emergency of international concern (PHEIC). Regardless of the outcome of the meeting, the risk of the outbreak is considered to be high.

According to a report, experts confirmed that the deadly outbreak originated from a wholesale animal market located in the central Chinese city of Wuhan.

According to a Xinhua news agency report cited on News.com.au, the scientists working with the Chinese Center for Disease Control and prevention revealed that the virus was initially transmitted from animals to humans during business transactions at the Huanan Seafood Wholesales market.

The market which has now been shuttered sold peacocks, rats, foxes, wolf pups, and other animals. The market had been earlier reported as the epicenter of the virus.

Thirty-three samples were collected from the western zone of the market where there was a concentration of wildlife trading. Thirty-one of the samples turned out to be positive when tested. The result confirmed everyone's fears that the outbreak was a result of wild animal trades in the market.

So far, the virus has infected 2,700 people, and 80 others have been killed by this virus.

As investigations are still ongoing on how to stop the spread of the virus, the Chinese government has temporarily placed a ban on the trading of wild animals. The government also promised to investigate and punish violators of the ban.

Where and when did Coronavirus COVID-19 start?

Widespread agreement on the origin of the coronavirus is believed to be December 2019 in a "wet market" in Wuhan where both dead and live animals (including fish and birds) are traded.

These markets put a increased risk of viruses moving from animals to people due to hygiene standards are difficult to maintain. Alive animals are hold and butchered on site. It is unknown the from which animal/s the latest Coronavirus is coming from. The host is thought to be bats. Although bats were not traded at the Wuhan market but may have infected other animals sold there.

The story of the Chinese doctor who tried to warn others about coronavirus

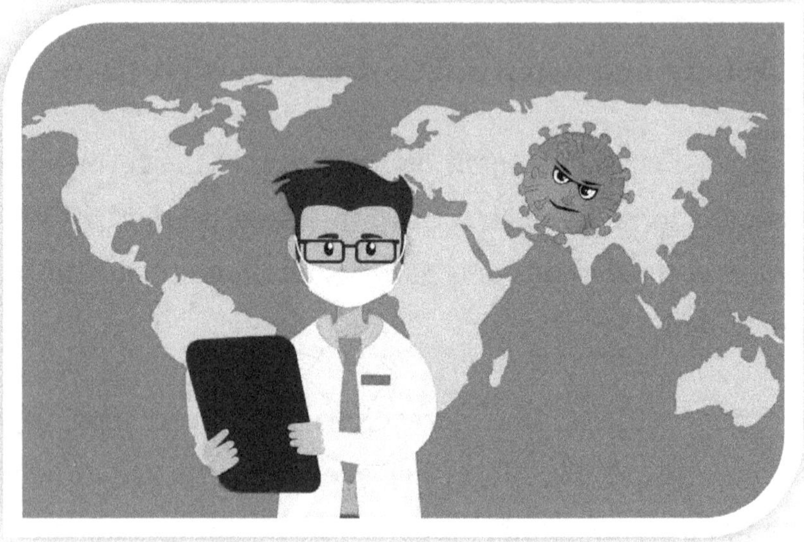

Dr Li Wenliang, who worked has ophthalmologist at Wuhan Central Hospital tried to warn fellow medical professionals about the outbreak at the end of December 2019. Apparently three days after the police warned him stop. He was then investigated for "spreading rumors". Dr. Li came back to work and caught the virus from a patient. Dr Li noted seven cases of a virus that he thought looked like SARS (the virus that led to a global epidemic in 2003). The 10th, January 2020 he began coughing, and then he had a fever and two days proximate he was in hospital. His parents also felt bad and were brought to hospital.

Ten days proximate, the 20th, January 2020, China declared the emergency outbreak.

Dr Li says was tested several times for coronavirus, all of them came back negative.

But On 30th January he posted again he tested positive. Dr Li died the 7th February 2020 in Wuhan, China.

The pathway of Covid-19

With thousands dead, cities of millions of people in China under lockdown, and countries closing their borders, not to mention travel bans to China has been like a game played by states all over the world to see who can issue theirs the fastest, it makes you wonder, "how did we get here?" "Where did this virus originate from, and how has it been able to spread so quickly?"

Here is a brief explanation of where this 'Demon virus' originated from; we shall also look at the pathway it has taken from the time of the first outbreak/patient zero up to this point where it has now become a global epidemic.

December 31, 2019: As countries all over the world are

preparing to usher in a new year, a good number of people in the Wuhan state of China report having pneumonia that has no clear origin. This report reaches the World Health Organization. On the same day, the hospitals discover that all the pneumonia patients have one thing in common: The Wuhan seafood market!

January 1, 2020: Authorities cordon off the Wuhan seafood market, suspecting it as the origin of the virus.

January 7, 2020: The Chinese authorities report that they have found the cause of the pneumonia-like condition. They declare it is a new virus that comes from the broader family of coronaviruses, and name it the coronavirus COVID-19.

January 9, 2020: China confirms the first coronavirus COVID-19 death. The number of infected people at this point stands at 40.

January 13, 2020: Thailand reports the first coronavirus case outside China.

January 15, 2020: Japan reports its first coronavirus case.

January 20, 2020: South Korea reports a coronavirus

case. On the same day, researchers discovered that the coronavirus could spread from one person to another. At this point, there were 282 cases of coronavirus reported in four countries.

January 21, 2020: Coronavirus reported cases rise to 314.

January 23, 2020: The reported cases increase to 581 cases, a majority of them being from China. The Government of Wuhan closes off the streets and shuts down public transportation.

January 30, 2020: The World Health Organization declares coronavirus COVID-19 a public health emergency; at this point, 18 countries outside China report 82 cases.

January 31, 2020: The coronavirus reaches every state in China, and in a period of 24-hours, authorities report 2,000 new cases. Reported cases now stand at 9,800 across 21 countries.

February 2, 2020: A 44 years old Chinese dies of coronavirus in the Philippines and becomes the first coronavirus death reported outside mainland China

February 4, 2020: Hong Kong reports the second death outside China.

February 17, 2020: According to WHO, the number of reported coronavirus cases stands at 71, 429. Of those, 70,635 cases are from China. The death toll is at 1775 globally, with only 3 of those deaths coming from countries outside China.

How Does The Coronavirus Spread?

The coronavirus is zoonotic. That means the virus is transmittable between animals and humans. In fact, the main hosts of coronaviruses are animals, which then transmit the virus either directly to you or through an intermediate animal. The evidence of that is in two earlier coronaviruses SARS and MERS.

According to discoveries, SARS is transmittable from civet cats to humans, but the virus first jumped from bats to civets, and so the civet was the intermediate carrier in that case.

MERS comes from dromedary camels to humans.

According to various reports, the outbreak of novel coronavirus jumped from bats to humans through an intermediate carrier that scientists are yet to determine.

Does The Coronavirus Spread From Human To Human?

The answer is yes; coronavirus can spread from one human to another through respiratory droplets. Respiratory droplets are the watery particles —saliva— that come out of your mouth or nose when you sneeze, cough, or breathe. If, for instance, you have coronaviruses and your respiratory droplets are in one way or another inhaled by a person near you, it shall infect the person. Researches have also confirmed asymptomatic transmission of the virus.

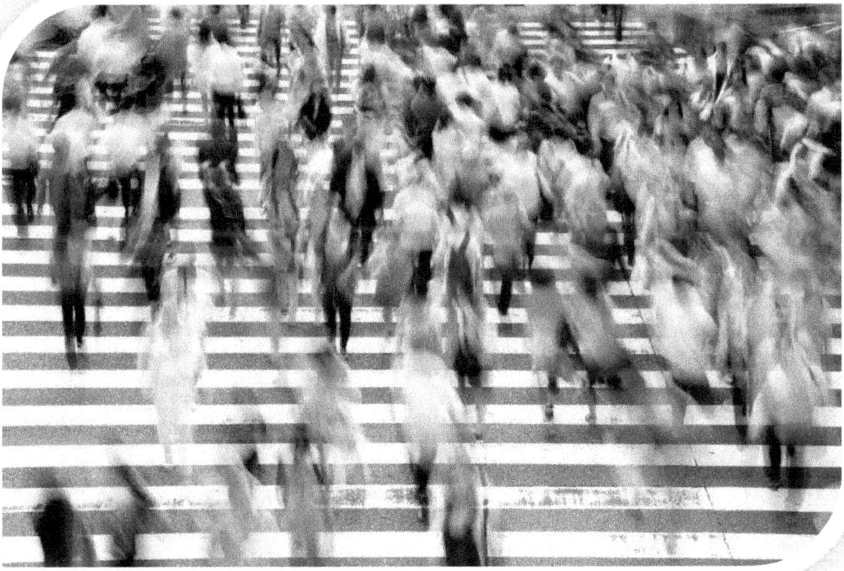

Additionally, if the person nearest to you also touches an object or an item that comes into contact with your respiratory droplets, they will get infected as well, especially if you used the same hands to touch your mouth or your face. Can We Lower the Risk Of Coronavirus From Humans-to-Humans?

Yes, we can, but only if you follow the recommended guidelines below.

- The standard recommendations for the prevention of the spread of coronavirus include;

- Washing your hands frequently

- Avoiding the habit of touching your mouth, eyes, and face.

- Disinfecting any object or surface you think you might come into contact with or are about to touch

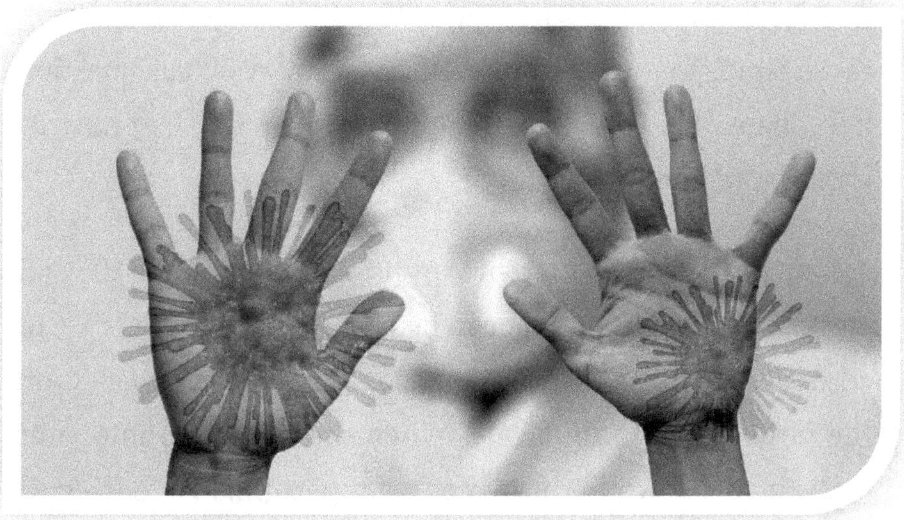

- Cook your meat and eggs thoroughly

- Avoid anyone with symptoms of coronavirus —we shall learn about symptoms shortly

- When coughing or sneezing, cover your mouth and nose

These guidelines will help you avoid coming into contact with infected respiratory droplets.

The Science of Coronaviruses

As you now know, coronaviruses can infect you when you

come into contact with the virus through an infected person's respiratory secretion like a sneeze and a cough, or through physically touching a surface that has the virus and then using those hands to touch your mouth, nose, or eyes. The question left unanswered is, "what happens when the coronavirus enters your body?"

One of the things that viruses have in common is they all carry genetic material that can be DNA or RNA. In the case of coronavirus, it has the RNA that contains all the information the virus needs to duplicate. When the virus gets into your body, it gets down to the process of replicating. Here it's how it does that.

What happens when the coronavirus gets into the body?

Once in your body, the coronaviruses bind themselves to the outer protein receptors of your cells and form what usually looks like a solar crown when viewed under an electron microscope. That image, matter of fact, is what gives the virus its name CORONA, which is a Latin word for crown.

When coronaviruses find relatable cells in your body, they pair up. If the outer layer of your cell were a lock, the outer layer of the coronavirus would be a key. If the key matches the lock, the lock will open. That is how the coronavirus opens up the right cell.

Once the virus gets into your cell, it accesses your cellular machinery. Usually, your body, and to be precise, your DNA, uses the cell machinery to produce proteins that serve different purposes in your body. When the coronavirus infects the cells, all that changes. The virus hijacks the machinery by releasing its RNA to the ribosome of the cell that is responsible for producing proteins, making it produce the proteins the virus needs to reproduce. This action automatically turns your cell into a factory of viruses. In short, the virus uses your cell machinery to duplicate. Once the production of viruses in your cells increases, they start migrating from the cell and damage it in the process. They then move to another cell and duplicate themselves again and keep repeating the cycle with all other cells.

Once your body detects the death of its cells, it triggers an immune response to fight the virus. The immune system sends cytokines that recruit immune cells and take them to the site of infection. The immune cells then fight off the viruses in a bid to restore order in the body.

This juncture is where the danger of coronavirus comes in. Here is how:

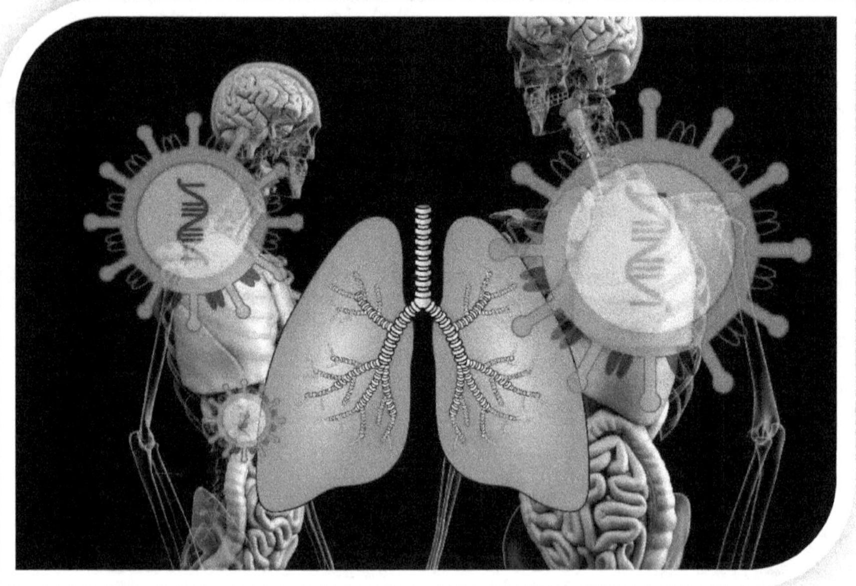

In a typical case, the immune response is usually safe and helpful to your body. That changes when a coronavirus attacks you. When your body notices an attack from a coronavirus, your immune response dispatches a massive number of cytokines to your lungs without regulation. That means your immune system launches an attack on your infected cells as well as your healthy ones.

The result of this cytokine-storm includes inflammation in your lungs, which causes fluids to leak through the air sacks. This process is what causes you to experience some of the mild symptoms like fever, cough headache, and being short of breath. When the situation gets worse, you experience severe symptoms like pneumonia and death.

Now that you know the facts about the novel coronavirus, we can discuss controversial coronavirus conspiracy theories and find out if they are true or false:

Who is most at risk?

Much like any other illness or coronavirus, elderly people have the highest health risk from 2019-nCoV. Young children are also at risk, as are those who are immunocompromised from existing conditions and medications.

On January 23, 2020, Chinese health officials announced that the death ratio of this illness heavily skewed toward

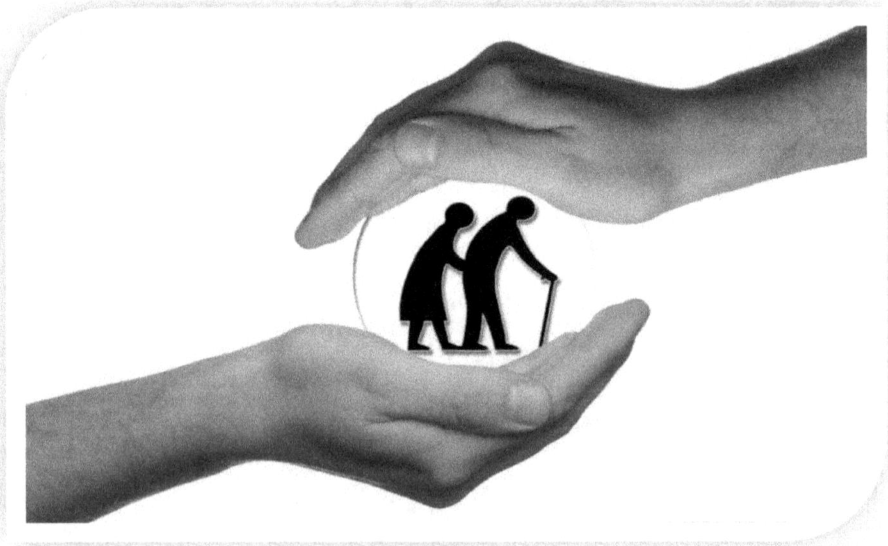

elderly men with pre-existing health conditions. Women and younger patients, including a young man who had no known health issues, have also perished at the hands of this virus. Therefore, despite there being higher risks factors for some patients, everyone who contracts the virus is at risk.

According to the New York Times, several medical experts involved with the SARS outbreak are heavily concerned about the current state of the 2019-nCoV.

Dr. Guan Yi from the University of Hong Kong said, "we have a chance to have a pandemic outbreak." After traveling to Wuhan in the hopes of helping out, Dr. Guan stated that he quickly left, feeling "powerless, very angry."

Columbia University epidemiologist Dr. W. Ian Lipkin reportedly advised the WHO and Chinese government officials that there's no good way to contain the spread of the disease. He was quoted as opining that "the horse is already out of the barn."

UPDATE (February 25, 2020):

The U.S. Centers for Disease Control and Prevention (CDC) and Canada's Chief Medical Officer of Health issued statements urging citizens to take precautions and begin preparing for a global pandemic.

In Canada, the statement said that people should stock up on non-perishable goods and prescription medications.

More information about this update – and how to prepare – is included proximate in this area.

THE SYMPTOMS

According to the World Health Organization, the common signs of coronavirus include breathing difficulties, shortness of breath, cough, and fever. However, these are signs of mild cases of infection. If you are in a severe case, the symptoms you will experience include organ failure, pneumonia, and even death.

That is how we got to where we are today.

Among various animals, coronaviruses can cause a variety of symptoms. While certain strains cause diarrhea in pigs and turkeys, infections are generally related to bad cold, resulting in mild to moderate-severe respiratory symptoms, such as runny nose and throat, fever, cough, shortness of breath, and difficulty breathing. In worse cases, influenza, severe acute respiratory syndrome, kidney failure and even death may cause infection.

Standard guidelines for preventing infection transmission include regular hand washing, coughing, and sneezing, shielding the mouth and nose, meat and eggs. Avoid near contact with people with respiratory symptoms such as coughing and sneezing.

Most coronaviruses spread like other cold-causing viruses: coughing and sneezing by infected people, touches of the hands or faces of the infected person, or touches such things as doorbells to which infected people have suffered.

At least once in your life, almost everyone receives a coronavirus infection, most often as a young child. Coronaviruses in the United States are more prevalent in autumn and winter, but everyone could be diagnosed with the coronavirus at any time.

Different Coronavirus Signs

The symptoms of most coronaviruses are similar to other high breathing illnesses, such as runny noses, coughing, sore throat, and fever at times.

You can do laboratory tests, including nose and throat samples and blood work, to figure out if you have a coronavirus in your cold, but there is no need to do so. The outcomes of the test would not affect the diagnosis of your symptoms.

Coronavirus vaccine

There is no coronavirus vaccine. To prevent infection by coronavirus, you do the same to prevent common cold: wash your hands vigorously with soap and warm water or a hand sanitizer made with alcohol.

Keep your hands and feet, nose and mouth, away from your eyes.

Avoid close contact with infected people.

You treat the same way you treat a coronavirus infection: have plenty of rest.

Drink water, drink the liquid.

Take medicine for a sore throat and fever. But don't offer ibuprofen or acetaminophen to children or teenagers under 19.

Moisturizer or steamy shower can also make the throat raw and scratchy.

In other nations, even though a coronavirus causes MERS or SARS, the type of coronavirus that is prevalent in the USA is not a serious threat to another healthy adult if you get ill, monitor and call the doctor if your symptoms get worse or if they don't go down.

Coronavirus symptoms are generally mild–including runny

nose, vomiting, nausea and fever–in some cases, they contribute to more serious diseases of the respiratory tract, including pneumonia and bronchitis. In older patients or people with existing health conditions, these can be particularly dangerous, and this appears to be the case with this novel coronavirus. Of the five early deaths, four have had underlying medical conditions that make them more vulnerable to the virus, as doctors further studied their medical history.

How far has it gone?

China bore the brunt of (so far) coronavirus infections. As of 31 January, over 11,900 cases and 259 deaths were registered by Chinese health authorities. Although the majority of cases are in the central province of Hubei, the disease spreads to Beijing, Shanghai, and Guangdong.

The maximum number of cases has been reported outside of China, Thailand, and Japan, with 14 people testing for the virus positively in each country. There are 13 incidents in Japan, 13 in South Korea, nine in Indonesia, eight in Malaysia, five in Vietnam, six in France and the United States.

The first two infections with coronavirus in the UK were confirmed on 31 January. The infected individuals came from the same household and were sick during their stay in a hotel in York. Work is underway to track who they might have been in contact with, although it is not thought that the hotel itself poses a significant infection risk. Eighty-three Britons rescued by the Foreign Office from Wuhan have been held for 14 days in quarantine.

In the USA, the Centers for Disease Control and Prevention recommended that there be no essential trips in China, while the United Kingdom Foreign and Commonwealth Office advises against travel to the province of Hubei and all but journeys critical to the rest of mainland China.

Although there are increasing cases in China, there is limited evidence of human-to-human transmission outside China. The first confirmed cases of human to human transmission in Europe were reported by a Chinese colleague visiting him in Shanghai in Germany on Tuesday, 28 January 2020. Also, people who have not traveled to China in Taiwan, Vietnam and Japan.

After the decision was initially delayed, the WHO declared an international public health emergency on 31 January 2020. General Director Tedros Adhanom Ghebreyesus listed, amongst the factors that contribute to the health agency's decision to announce an international emergency, the incidence of disease in China and the cases of human-to-human infection outside of China.

Since 2009 only five international public health emergencies have been reported: the swine flu pandemic in 2009, the polio outbreak in 2014, Ebola in 2014 in Western Africa, Zika in 2015, and Ebola widespread in the Democratic Republic of the Congo in 2019.

Nevertheless, other forms of coronaviruses are severe. Approximately 858 people died of the respiratory syndrome (MERS), which first emerged in Saudi Arabia in 2012 and then in other Middle East, Africa, Asia and Europe. The first American to be treated with MERS was in Indiana in April 2014 and another outbreak in Florida was confirmed. Both had come back from Saudi Arabia just now. The outbreak of MERS in Korea was the most significant outside of the Arab Peninsula in May 2015. In 2003, a severe acute respiratory syndrome (SARS) epidemic resulted in 774 deaths. There were no further records of SARS cases as of 2015.

By early 2020, however, after an epidemic by China in December 2019, the World Health Organization reported a new type of new coronavirus in 2019 (2019-nCoV).

Coronavirus also causes symptoms of upper respiratory infections, such as the stuffy nose, cough and sore throat. You should handle them with medications for rest and on - the-counter. Coronavirus can also cause infections of the middle ear in infants.

The Erasmus Medical Center has been identified as the first hCov-EMC classified as Human Coronavirus in mid-2012. 5 out of the 11 reported patients of this deadly disease have died; this highly mutant strain of coronavirus is exceptionally lethal. This mutated virus is identical to that found in bat species of coronavirus. Sadly, this new and deadly virus has sprung from animals to humans, and, more troublingly, a human to human transmission has taken place recently.

The first recorded victim was identified in June 2002 when a 60-year-old male was found to have influenza symptoms and difficulty breathing in a Jidda Saudi Arabia Hospital. Within a few days of hospital admission, this patient was killed by kidney failure and severe pneumonia. There have been 11 more cases over the past seven months, including one in England at the beginning of 2013. This case was particularly disturbing for international infectious disease scientists as well as for the WHO, as it seems that the British victim contracted his father, who has recently traveled to the Middle East with the new and deadly coronavirus. The virus's apparent ability to quickly spring from animal to human is alarming.

Influenza, like fever, cough, and difficulty breathing, is signs of Cov-EMC infection that quickly progresses into extreme pneumonia and renal failure. The international community has issued a warning to all medical institutions and physicians to be aware of any suspected respiratory infections and to notify them.

I was coughing. Have I got this virus?

If you haven't visited Wuhan recently, China, or have close contact with someone who is sick who recently visited Wuhan, China, you will rarely have this infection. Nonetheless, it is normal to be anxious— and there are ways to reduce the anxiety, such as calming yourself or putting threats in perspective.

When you live in the US, you have much more flu or the common cold. It is still the flu season, so elevated influenza incidence will not disappear in the near future. Tell your doctor about your symptoms if you feel sick and have been in Wuhan, China, or have close contact with someone who has it.

How can I guard myself?

Based on what we know so far, the same precautions you can take (and should take) to shield you from flu: wash your hands, close your mouth when you cough, and stay away from sick people.

How does China try to stop the virus?

The officials in Wuhan shut down all transport in the area, home to more than 11 million residents, on January 22, 2020. Busses and subways were suspended and all flights and trains canceled in and out of the area.

Nevertheless, others were not sure whether these quarantines would be effective: "It's the science that seeks to control the 11 million-strong population," said Gauden Galea, the representative of the World Health Organization in China, to the Associated Press. "It was not used before as a test of public health. At this stage, we can't say it will or won't. "Main towns across the country have canceled Lunar New Year celebrations, an enormous holiday in China.

With confirmed SARS-COV2 infections, the reported diseases ranged from people with mild symptoms to people who are seriously ill and dying. Symptoms can include Fever, cough, and shortness of breath.

The distribution of SARS-COV-2 infection in China and worldwide is explained in the following study. According to the first official declaration by the Wuhan Municipal Health Commission, viral pneumonia (proximate confirmed as

SARS-COV2 -related pneumonia) was diagnosed in 27 patients by December 31, 2019.

All cases occurred in, including Wuhan, Hubei, China. Seven severe cases, but no deaths were reported. As of January 10, 2020, the number of confirmed cases in 2019 SARS-COV2 infection in Wuhan rose to 41, with 1 death reported.

Ten days proximate, on January 20, 2020, 16 the number of infected cases increased to 217, including 198 in Wuhan, 14 in Guangdong, and 5 in Beijing. In addition, four cases outside of China were confirmed (Thailand / Japan / South Korea).

The number of confirmed cases increased rapidly from January 20, 2020, to 440, with 9 deaths by January 21, 2020; 571 with 17 deaths until January 22, 2020; 830 with 25 deaths by January 23, 2020; and 1287 with 41 deaths by January 24, 2020. From the last report on January 25, 2020, a total of 1975 patients from 30 provinces (autonomous regions and municipalities) were confirmed with the infection with SARS-COV-2 on the Chinese mainland, with a total 56 deaths.

The latest mortality rate was approximately 2.84%, with a total of 2684 additional suspected cases.

In addition, 23 cases outside of China confirmed (Thailand,

Singapore, Malaysia, France, the United States, Japan, South Korea, Vietnam, Nepal, Australia) dated January 25, 2020.

China National Health Commission stated the details of the first 17 deaths by January 22, 2020, including 13 men and 4 women.

The median death age was 75 (range 48-89) years. Before admission, 11 cases with other diseases were complicated, and 5 had a surgical history. Fever (64.7%) and cough (52.9%) were the more frequent first symptoms.

The mean number of days from the first symptom to death was 14.0 (range 6-41) and tended to be shorter in people aged 70 years (11.5 [range 6-19] days) than in people under 70 years (20 [area 10]) 41 days; P = 0.033).

Research has shown that the novel virus has spread rapidly in China since the Wuhan Municipal Health Commission first officially announced on December 31, 2019.

The infection has spread between January 20, 2020, and January 25, 2020, according to the National Health Commission Increase very quickly. The detection and reporting of the infection may have become more important as it has been reported nationwide.

It has been also showed that the COVID-19 had caused a

total of 1975 infections and 56 deaths in 26 days since the first official announcement. The current COVID-19 mortality is around 2.84%, which is lower than that of 9, 6% of the SARS CoV, which spread to 30 countries/regions worldwide, infected 8098 people and killed 774 patients25 from November 2002 to July 2003 and less than 34.4% of the MERS-CoV, which spread to 27 countries/regions worldwide spread, infected 2494 people and killed 858 patients from September 2012 to September 2019.

However, in the first three months from November 2002 to February 2003, in Guangdong, China, only one diagnosis of atypical pneumonia, originally known as Chlamydia pneumonia, was viewed (lproximate confirmed to be caused by SARS) 5 deaths. Taken together, these facts show that current mortality is lower than that of the SARS-CoV and the MERS-CoV, but the COVID-19 appears to be very contagious.

The first deaths occurred mainly in the elderly. Despite the fact that most of them had comorbidities or a history of surgery prior to admission, the possible association between the underlying medical conditions and the death associated with COVID-19 was not clear. For SARS, it has been reported that the average duration of first symptoms until hospital admission 3, 8 days, and the admission to death was 17.4 days for deaths.

The study also found that people over 70 years had shorter mean days (11.5 days). The first symptom of death than those under 70 years (20 days) shows that older people may progress faster than younger people.

Similar results were found for SARS in that the average time from admission to death was 5.7 days for those aged 80 to 93 years, 9.4 days for those aged 60 to 79 years, and over 12.0 Days for people under the age of 60. It was also reported that older age (> 60 years) was a risk factor that correlated with mortality in MERS. Although a clear comparison was not possible, the public should refer to the elderly that may be less vulnerable to COVID-19.

Coronaviruses During Pregnancy

This newly recognized coronavirus, which causes a disease called COVID-19, is spreading rapidly across China, crossing international borders to infect people in neighboring countries, and people infected with the virus are traveling to other continents via commercial airlines. SARS-COV-2 will certainly infect pregnant women, though the question remains whether the coronavirus disease 2019 will have a similar or different effect on them compared to SARS-CoV and MERS-CoV.

In order to investigate the possible obstetric consequences of infection for mother and child, this communication describes the current state of knowledge about the effects of other coronavirus infections in pregnancy.

Pneumonia during Pregnancy

Pneumonia due to an infectious etiology is an important cause of morbidity and mortality in pregnant women.

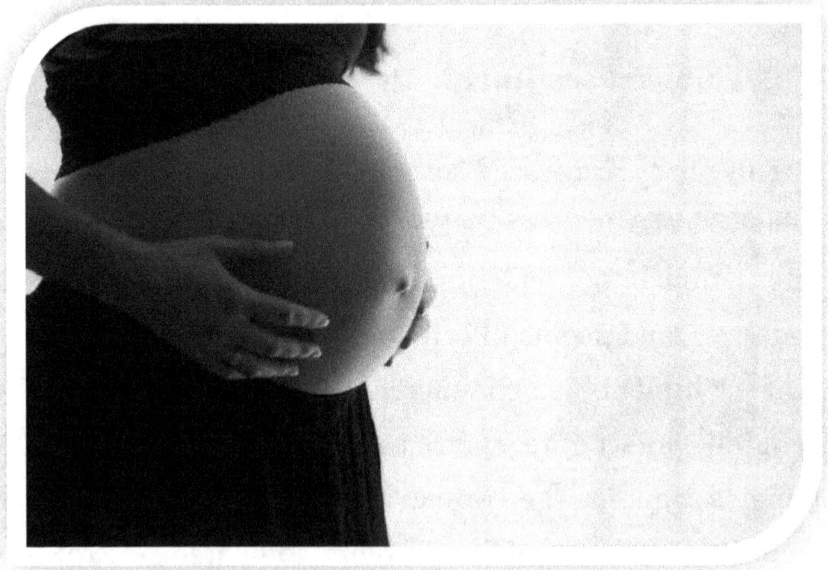

It is the most common non-obstetric infectious disease that occurs during pregnancy. In one study, pneumonia was the third leading cause of indirect maternal death. About 25

percent of pregnant women who develop pneumonia must be hospitalized in intensive care units and require ventilation support.

Although bacterial pneumonia is a serious disease if it occurs in pregnant women, even if the active substances are susceptible to antibiotics, viral pneumonia has an even higher level of morbidity and mortality during pregnancy.

As with other infectious diseases, the normal physiological changes in the mother associated with pregnancy - including changes in cell-mediated immunity and changes in lung function - have been shown to affect both susceptibility to and clinical severity of pneumonia.

This was historically evident in earlier epidemics. The mortality rate (CFR) in pregnant women infected with influenza during the 1918-1919 pandemic was 27% - even higher when exposure occurred in the third trimester and over 50% when pneumonia occurred.

During the Asian flu epidemic of 1957–1958, 10% of all deaths occurred in pregnant women, and their CFR was twice as high as that of infected women who were not pregnant. The most common undesirable obstetric consequences of pneumonia in mothers for all reasons are premature membrane rupture (PROM) and premature birth (PTL), intrauterine fetal death (IUFD), intrauterine growth restriction (IUGR) and death of the newborn.

GLOBAL EMERGENCY?

According to a statement released by WHO on the 30th of January, the outbreak has been classified as a global health emergency.

This health emergency alert was to spur countries around the world into action by coordinating their

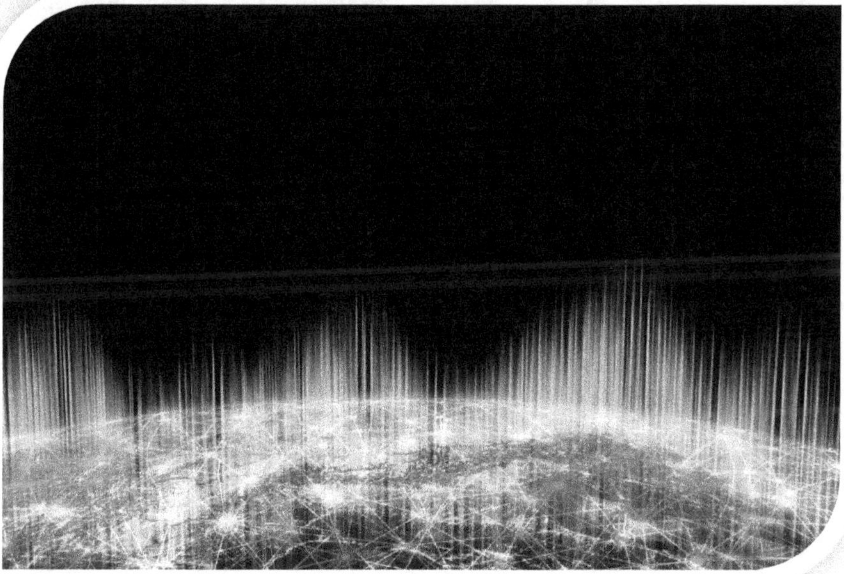

response according to the guidance of the United Nations health agency.

This type of global emergency has been announced five times since 2005. These calls were made in the following instances - swine flu (2009), polio (2014), Ebola (2014), Zika (2016), and Ebola (2019).

Transmission Of The Virus

Several researches have been carried out as to how coronavirus spreads from one human to the other. These researches have affirmed that the contraction of this infection occurs from the transmission of secreted fluid from the respiratory system. Coronavirus can be contracted through the following ways;

- Reckless sneezing and coughing without covering the mouth. This can disperse droplets that are capable of transmitting the virus into the air.

- Shaking and touching an infected person.

- Coming in contact with an infected surface, then touching your eyes or nose with the same unwashed hands.

- On rare occasions, coronavirus can also be spread through contact with feces.

People living in the United States are more vulnerable to

this disease during the fall and winter. Regardless of this, the disease is still active during the rest of the year. Young people are more vulnerable to contracting this disease. Most humans will be infected with at least one coronavirus in their lifetime. Coronavirus is so contagious because of its mutating abilities. In order to prevent transmission, stay at home, and rest when exhibiting any of the symptoms of these symptoms. Strictly avoid contact with other people too. Also, remember to cover your nose and mouth with a tissue or handkerchief while coughing or sneezing. Make sure to dispose of used tissues in order to maintain proper hygiene in the home.

The World Health Organization (WHO) issued a global public health emergency alert for only the sixth time in its history on January 30, 2020.

Per the WHO, the group has to agree via a vote that there's "an extraordinary event which is determined to constitute a public health risk to other States through the international spread of disease and to potentially require a coordinated international response."

The WHO was founded in 1948 but did not use the global public health emergency designation until 2009. Here's a quick look at the other five outbreaks that were deemed serious enough to demand a global public health emergency alert.

- 2009 Swine Flu pandemic (affected 11-21 percent of the world's population; killed between 151,000 – 579,000).
- 2014 Polio Infection (359 new cases of polio were diagnosed in Cameroon, Pakistan, Syria, etc.).
- 2014 Ebola epidemic (affected an estimated 28,630 people; killed 11,315 people in West Africa).
- 2016 Zika virus (estimates show that somewhere between 497,000 and 1.48 million were likely affected worldwide; total death count still isn't known).
- 2018 Ebola epidemic, although the WHO did not declare it a public health emergency until 2019 (Still ongoing

in the Congo; 3,300+ cases; 2,200 deaths).

The outbreak, which the World health organization has referred to as an international Public Health concern, has triggered research, funding and action from health agencies across the globe, countries and governments, as well as private and personal efforts. The WHO has said that the sum of 675 million dollar for preparedness and response plan would need to be launched. This plan would cover the months of February through April.

Also, In China, the government has put immigration measures in place to ease the entry of non-governmental organizations willing to come in and offer assistance in the fight against the outbreak. Humanitarian relief organizations such as Project HOPE have indicated interest in working through existing health systems and agencies in China. The relief organization has supplied over 2 million face masks, 11,000 protective suits and 280,000 pairs of exam gloves to public hospitals in Wuhan with a further 365,000 face masks which was also provided to the Shanghai children's medical center. Another organization which has shown its support is Direct Relief. They have so far delivered 572,000 N95 respirator masks and over 340,000 gloves as well as other items such as shoe covers.

The USAID delivered protective gears to Laos. Save The

Children Fund delivered 36,000 face masks to Indonesian hospitals and to Wuhan. Mèdecin Sans Frontieres has also offered to support health authorities in mainland China and Hong Kong.

Other companies with no direct involvement with the items needed for protection in the care for patients have lent support by other means. For example, the hospitals constructed in Wuhan over 10 days had beds supplied to it. It also made power supply guaranteed in certain facilities with network cables channeled to facilities as well as the installation of 5G remote video diagnostic centers which has enabled medical staff to carry out diagnostic procedures on suspected patients remotely.

Another strategy than has been of help is the fight of misinformation. Companies like Baidu and Qihoo 360 have set up platforms on their apps that help users know in real-time the locations of confirmed and suspected cases of the virus. This information helps travelers in avoiding the affected regions and further reducing any potential of spread. Others like Tencent' "Mepedia" and Ping An's "AskBob" are artificial intelligence programs that serve as remote doctors in answering questions and providing verified information on preventive and protective protocols to its users. Because of the economic devastating effect of the thousands of people who have had to miss work because of the quarantine measures in place, other platforms have come up with ideas to help a lot of people work from home. These platforms include Alibaba's DingTalk, Tencent's WeChatWork and Meeting, ByteDance's Feishu and Huawei's WeLink. Such platforms have added features such as video conferences and call time, online check-ins and industry-specific solutions.

On the aspect of education, schools are closed all over China to prevent further and faster spread of the virus. However, it's now easier for people to undertake classes and courses online. Online education platforms like Liulishuo, Onion Academy and Zuoyebang are offering free classes to students online, nationwide. Lecturers and university professors are not left out also as they can now conduct online classes to a wide range of their students who can attend these classes online from the comfort and safety of their homes.

Tech solutions are also being offered to aid speedier diagnosis and treatment. Software's with AI computing capabilities, RNA predicting algorithms, high tech CT scanners, AI imaging, cloud platforms and remote advanced post-procession software's are being made available to hospitals in Wuhan.

On the flip side, the global nature and approach to the corona virus outbreak has also brought about fringes in administration, political and diplomatic frictions. In the following weeks after the outbreak, questions and controversies have trailed the travel ban placed on Chinese citizens. This brings to mind the dilemma that surrounded the Ebola outbreak of 2014-2016 in which prohibitions were put in place to stall travelers from west African countries, which was a violation of the IHR (International Health Regulations).

The widespread use of quarantine has also been a topic of controversy. The city of Wuhan was placed on cordon sanitaire, an unprecedented action. The 11 million inhabitants of the city have been totally barred from entering or leaving the city and on a larger scale, 760 million people across the country have been restricted and in some form of residential lockdown. There is a mental side effect to this which many people have argued for and against. Other countries like the United States of America, Australia have also imposed some form of quarantine or the other and immigration processes have been under close monitoring . The WHO has however, been silent on the above quarantine measures and the outcry they have raised.

The Impact of the COVID-19 outbreak on the cruise industry

Due to the peculiarities of cruise travel, which essentially brings a large number of persons together in close proximity, the risk of spread of infectious diseases are particularly high in such situations. This was seen in the case of the Diamond Princess Cruise ship which had embarked on a holiday trip to Yokohama, Japan that was to morph into a deadly nightmare. About 3,711 cruise passengers and crew members were caught in the disease outbreak, and about 621 of them were confirmed to carry the virus. After a prolonged quarantine that drew mixed criticisms from international quarters regarding the handling of cruise ships, over a thousand of the passengers were allowed to leave the ill-fated ship, but not before two of the infected passengers had died.

The criticism was largely as a result of existing cruise travel regulations which view passengers on board ships as being outside of national borders and hence, giving countries the freedom to either accept or reject their docking. Such measures may be seen to rather than control infection spread, actually worsen it. In some other cases, this might seem to be the prudent step to take. An example is seen in the Holland America's Wester dam cruise ship which several countries rejected even with no reports on board of any cases of the virus, and which would proximate be accepted by Cambodia, a decision they may have regretted as proximate was reported that one of the passengers tested positive for the virus. This regret however, may have been fortunately short-lived as the US CDC proximate confirmed that the passenger did not have the virus and indeed, neither did any of the other passengers.

Ports are refusing to take in cruise ships which have been either to Chinese ports or which have on board, Chinese passengers. As well as enhanced screening and medical evaluation for persons who display symptoms of the disease. As the Wuhan coronavirus continues to spread outside China, the world health organization has declared it as a global emergency. "*An extraordinary event*" that concerns public health is termed "*public health emergency of international concern*" (PHEIC) by the world health organization (who).

- Is the outbreak unusual or unexpected? For the 2019-NCoV - a never-before-seen virus, the answer is yes.

- Is the outbreak risky to more than one country? The answer is also yes since there have been dozens of exported cases on four continents.

- Does the outbreak require a "coordinated international response"? Again, the answer is yes since airport screenings and aid money are needed to limit the spread of the virus.

WHO's official definition says, "*An outbreak is considered a PHEIC when the situation is serious, unusual or unexpected.*" there is an emergency committee of the International Health Regulations (IHR) that convenes to discuss the situation. Members of the committee are health experts from 196 countries including all who member states who've agreed to its current revision in 2005. The director-general takes the final decision after assessing evidence including human-to-human transmission rates.

The Frequency at Which WHO Denote Outbreaks as PHEIC

Since the term was coined, that who has made such a declaration roughly once every two years? However, the WHO weighs up the economic risks and the impact on industries such as tourism affects the WHO's decision before declaring public health emergencies. The regulations seek to "avoid unnecessary interference with international traffic and trade." there has been criticism at who for being too slow or too quick to declare a global health emergency. After the outbreak of SARS and h5n1 (bird flu) in the early 2000s, who developed procedures to declare a PHEIC and implemented these procedures in 2005. Since then, six emergencies have been declared.

They are listed here from the newest to the oldest.

- The Wuhan coronavirus (starting at the end of 2019)
- The current Ebola outbreak in the democratic republic of Congo (2019)
- The Zika virus (2016)
- Polio (2014)

- West Africa's Ebola outbreak (2014-2016)

- H1N1 virus (popularly called a strain of "swine flu"). It caused an influenza pandemic (2009)

The WHO took a year after the outbreak of Ebola in the democratic republic of Congo before declaring it a PHEIC.

The Meaning of the PHEIC Status

The main benefit of declaring an outbreak as a PHEIC is that it boosts public health measures, increases funding and resources available to prevent or reduce international spread. While the WHO tries not to cause trade restrictions, common measures include airport screening of passengers and other recommendations on trade and travel. The emphasis of these, who to manage PHEIC situations is to contain the outbreak at its origin. Also, countries must be transparent with the information concerning outbreak and possibly, isolate infected patients.

Why This Virus Is Considered a Pandemic?

As argue in the earlier topic, WHO has declared the 2019-NCoV virus as a global health emergency? But does it qualify as a pandemic? Find out by analyzing some epidemiology basics argue in this branch. Recall the town where you grew up and the popular infections back then. Then, you will discover that an "endemic" level of disease is never zero. Examples, malaria in some African countries or chickenpox in the United States. The truth is, endemic should be expected but never preferable. The onset of an outbreak can be a sudden increase in the number of people with a specific disease within a small geographical region. It can also be the start of a unique disease like the never-been-seen-before strain of the flu. An outbreak becomes an epidemic once it expands to a broader population. Hence, novel coronavirus qualifies as an epidemic (re-read the earlier topic about whose criteria for assigning an outbreak as a PHEIC).

However, epidemics can be severe and predominantly affect one region (in this case, China) without ever becoming a pandemic. According to the center for disease control and prevention, a pandemic is one that has affected a large number of people across several countries or continents. When classifying an epidemic as a pandemic, the severity of

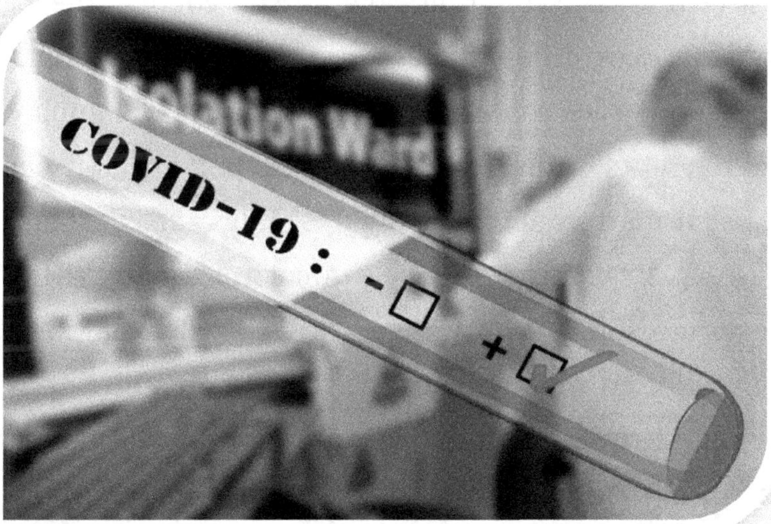

illnesses and the number of deaths are never considered. For example, if there are 39 confirmed coronavirus cases in Japan, 32 confirmed cases in Singapore and 29 in Thailand, but there are 28,000 cases in China. Then, the virus can't be considered a pandemic yet. Hence, based on the current number of confirmed cases, the Wuhan coronavirus is not yet a pandemic. The prospect of it becoming a pandemic looks increasingly likely as scientists learn more about the virus. Since this coronavirus is readily transferrable between humans, it is more of influenza (a standard pandemic agent) than other coronaviruses.

It can also be called a pandemic provided the number of cases in Europe and the United States continue to escalate drastically. Apart from the case count, the global consequences differentiate a pandemic from an epidemic. Right now, a few countries face real health or economic crises, but the hit to China's workforce is steep. It's mostly business as usual apart from the airport screenings and constant hand-washing. By comparison, the coronavirus causing the Middle Eastern respiratory syndrome (MERS) is less severe. It has only affected approximately 2,500 people since it started circulating in humans in 2012. Most of the affected persons are in and around the Arabian Peninsula. In contrast, the coronavirus responsible for the severe acute respiratory syndrome (SARS) is considered a pandemic. Why? It has not only affected 26 countries (especially across China, in Canada, Vietnam, Singapore, Taiwan, and Hong Kong), it continues to propagate across various regions and continents.

This new coronavirus could be similar to H1N1 swine flu that caused a pandemic in 2009. The H1N1 swine flu virus keeps circulating as one of the main strains of the seasonal flu despite subsidence in its outbreak since 2010.

TAKE ACTION

If you think you may have it, wear a surgical mask (especially when in public). Consult your doctor or a recognized health practitioner for medical advice. Masks serve a public health benefit in reducing transmission because it limits the volume and travel distance of expiratory droplets dispersed when coughing, sneezing or

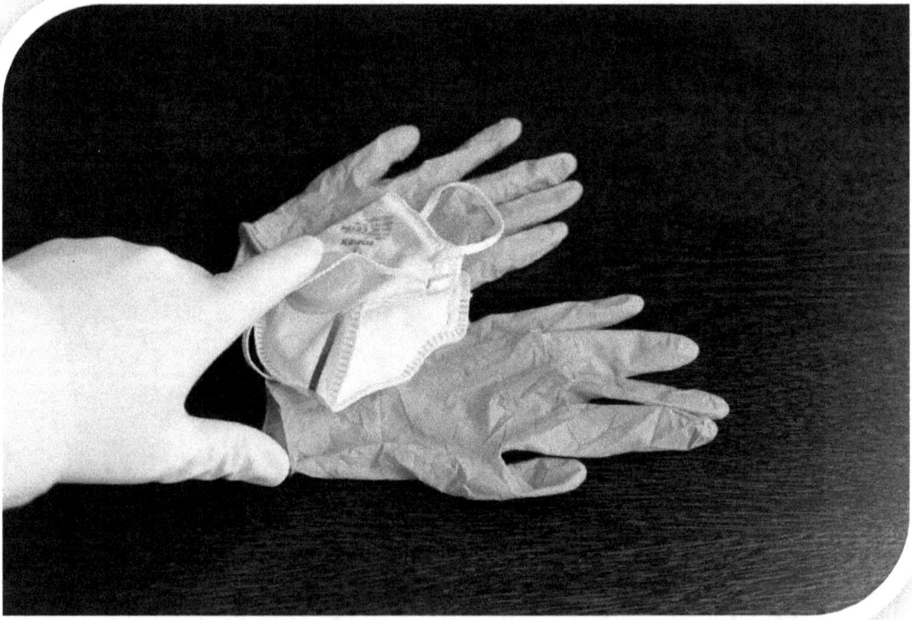

talking. When masks are unavailable, use a tissue or a flexed elbow to cover a cough or sneeze. Then, discard the tissue in the trash and wash your hands immediately.

Note: ineffective methods include eating garlic, gargling with mouthwash and rinsing the nose.

The Best Practices for Putting On the Mask

- Carefully place masks to cover the mouth and nose. Then, tie securely to reduce gaps between the mask and the face. Also, don't touch the mask while it's in use.

- Untie the lace from the back to remove the mask

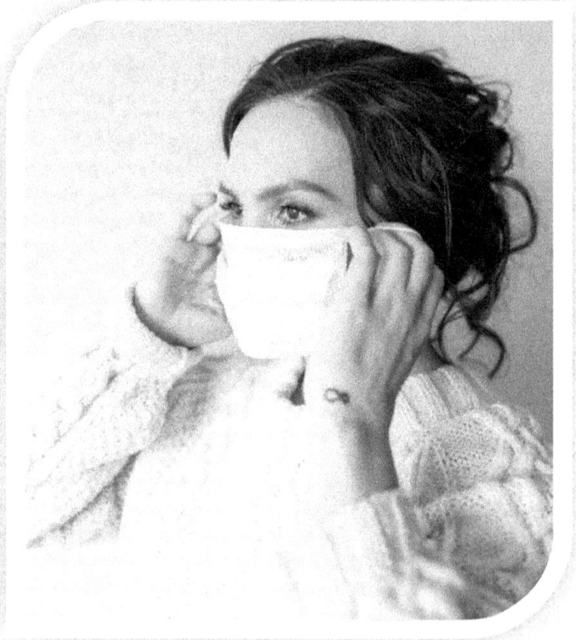

- If you touch the masks unwittingly, clean your hands with soap and water or an alcohol-based hand rub.

- Once mask become damp, replace with a new clean and

dry one

- Do not re-use masks. Dispose of masks after use or upon removal immediately

Other actions you should take are:

- Seek medical attention at once. But call the doctor ahead and follow his instructions before going to his office

- Don't be in physical contact with other people and stay at home to get medical help. If you don’t stay alone, isolate yourself from other people in your home and use a separate bathroom

- Cancel all your travel plans

- Stop sharing household items such as dishes, writing implements or towels.

- Health officials are urging vigilance since much is still unknown about the Wuhan coronavirus outbreak. But where traveling is compulsory, you must exercise preventive measures to avoid contracting the virus.

- Here's how travelers can protect themselves from this outbreak:

- Avoid close contact with people exhibiting cold

symptoms.

- The most common symptoms of those who contracted the Wuhan virus are sore throat, headaches, chills, and fever. Difficulty in breathing is less common. Also, avoid getting in contact with people displaying symptoms of pneumonia or common colds like runny noses or coughing.

- Wearing a mask is less effective than washing your hands regularly

- While many people have lined up to purchase face masks, it does little to protect anyone's health. Except for healthcare providers, wearing masks have never an effective way to protect yourself from infectious diseases. Also, scrub your hands for at least 20 seconds.

- Steer clear of live animals while in China

- Though scientists are not yet sure which animal spread the virus to people, they have traced the Wuhan virus to a local seafood market with live animals. New evidence suggests that horseshoe bats are likely responsible for transmitting the SARS virus to humans. Since the SARS incidence (some eighteen years ago), there have been repeated calls to improve or close down live animal markets in China. However, the recent evidence proves that live animal markets are a threat to the general public health and especially, those who work in them.

- Report your symptoms to a health authority

- Immediately you become ill after coming back from China, report your symptoms to your doctor or certified health practitioner. Don't forget to inform them about your travel history. However, restricting travel in areas with known cases of the virus won't be effective. Once you start getting sick when being screened at the airport, you might be isolated to avoid transmitting the disease.

- Lastly, travelinsurance.com states that most standard trip cancelation insurance policies do not cover virus outbreak. Also, if you hold an existing travel insurance policy,

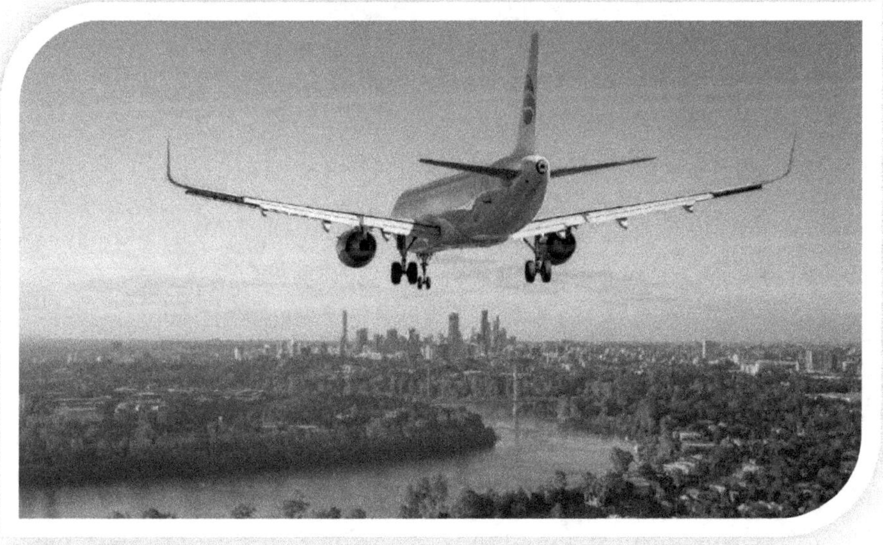

contact your travel insurance providers to know whether or not any of their plans have any coverage.

In 98% of the cases the symptoms are same as the normal flu virus symptoms like fever cough and cold but in case the person is having low immunity it will have severe symptoms like pneumonia thus extreme of ages like old age and children less than 5 years are at the risk.

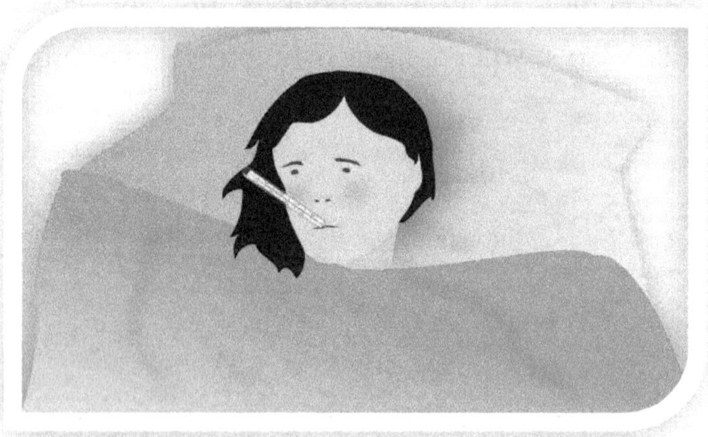

In case you have the fever cough and cold then don't panic the important expect is that if you have recent international travel history or you have been in contact with the person who is been diagnosed as positive or maybe you have been in contact with the person who had recently travelled to the international places then you should get yourself tested.

As there is no vaccine available for prevention at the moment, the best way of protecting oneself is by minimizing exposure to the virus. Protection guidelines are the established, are for all respiratory diseases and are as follows:

Avoid contact with people who are ill as much as possible.

Stay at home when you are ill to avoid spreading the virus to others.

Don’t touch your face with contaminated hands. Viruses can easily gain access into your system via mucosa such as your eyes, mouth, and nostrils.

Disinfection of household objects should be carried out routinely especially if there is a sick person in the home.

Cover your sneeze or cough with a tissue and discard that tissue afterwards to avoid reintroducing the shed viruses into your body system.

Hand washing with soap or an alcohol-based hand sanitizer as frequently as possible and especially after using the bathroom or before eating. Hand sanitizers should be used when water and soap aren't readily available. But hand washing remains the preferred means of hand hygiene.

Wearing of face mask is only recommended for people who are manifesting symptoms of COVID-19.

Wearing of face masks by people who are otherwise well has not been shown to have much benefits but rather, may have a paradoxical effect. Face masks are not meant to be worn on a long term basis, and definitely not meant to be re-used. Doing this may predispose one to a respiratory infection arising from a cocktail of trapped dust and nasal mucus secretions, humid and warm air which creates a favorable medium for growth of microorganisms. Falling sick would then further reduce the individual's immunity to the coronavirus.

Healthy people don’t need to wear facemasks for prevention, even in an area where coronavirus is prevalent. Following general measures like avoiding exposure, hand washing, maintenance of respiratory hygiene is more important than wearing a facemask to reduce transmission of disease. Also, healthy individuals who are taking care of coronavirus infected persons should wear a facemask when in the same room with them.

Even for countries where the risk of infection is low, there is need for every person to take necessary precautionary measures on their side to prevent this public health threat. Some of these measures are listed below:

With approach of the flu season, everyone should get the flu vaccine and take other hygienic measures to minimize the spread of illness. They may also consider taking antiviral flu medications if the doctor prescribes them. These drugs have been shown to not only reduce the severity of disease, but also shorten its duration.

Healthcare providers should be vigilant and aware enough to protect themselves while treating coronavirus infected patients.

Healthcare providers should be able to able to identify a person who has a specific history (travel to china, fever, respiratory symptoms) and take appropriate steps as needed.

If a person has traveled to China recently or has in some way been exposed to coronavirus infected patients, they should limit their activities and movement. Specific instructions and guidelines should be followed to ensure that they play their role in preventing the transmission of disease. If they develop COVID-19 symptoms, then they should notify the relevant health authorities and ask for medical assistance.

Pregnant women

Women undergo immunological and physiological changes during pregnancy that might make them more vulnerable to infections, including COVID 19. The evidence of COVID 19 causing severe illness in pregnant women is not present, but it is supported by the fact that other forms of coronavirus more severe illness in pregnant women as compared to the general population. Pregnant women are advised to follow the general health guidelines to reduce the risk of infection.

Many viral infections can cause adverse fetal outcomes as reported in influenza, SARS-CoV-1, and MERS-CoV infection. It may therefore be deduced that COVID-19 infections during pregnancy may be involved in adverse fetal outcomes due to the similarities in makep. Pregnant women with COVID-19 infections experience less adverse maternal and fetal complications as compared to pregnant women with SARS-CoV-1 infection however.

Even though there have been two cases of neonatal COVID 19 so far, these have occurred in the presence of close contact with infected persons and there is still a lack of sufficient evidence to support a vertical transmission of the SARS-CoV-2 virus which is transmission occurring from mother to child through the placenta during pregnancy, perinatally through contact with the mother's body fluids during delivery, or through the breast milk during breastfeeding.

Precautions for pregnant women:

Pregnant women should be considered a high-risk population for coronavirus infection.

Health education and screening facilities should be made readily available for women.

Newborns with suspected or confirmed infection should be isolated, and should not be breastfed.

Following the WHO general guidelines like hand washing, avoiding contact exposure, avoiding exposure with dead animals, etc.

School Children

The number of children affected by the COVID 19 infections is few as compared to adults. The reason is unknown, but it may be due to a difference in the immune system of age groups. Parents and teachers should encourage children to follow hygienic measures to protect themselves from the disease.

Some parents have opted to keep their children at home while many schools in China especially in the Hubei province of Wuhan have remained closed even with the end of the holiday season.

International Travel and Health

If a person is planning to travel, they should check the travel advisories. Consult your doctor before traveling if you are suffering from any health conditions which make you more vulnerable to respiratory infections.

The CDC recommends avoiding non-essential travel to China, and if you must travel:

Avoid close contact with people who are sick.

Avoid coming in close contact with animals whether alive or dead. Also keep away from animal markets and wild farms and their products.

Wash hands frequently, each session lasting at least 20 seconds and using soap and water. Alcohol-based hand sanitizers can be made use of in the absence of soap and water.

Older adults and travelers with underlying health issues may be at risk for more severe disease.

On the 10th of January 2020, WHO issued the first report on travel advice concerning the outbreak of new coronavirus in China. According to the report, as the mode of transmission of the virus was not yet fully established, travelers were advised to adhere to general health practices to reduce the spread of respiratory infections.

Health providers are also enjoined to give health education to travelers about disease symptoms and prevention. If a traveler exhibits the signs and symptoms of respiratory disease, health authorities should be notified and the contact details of the traveler is taken for follow up. WHO did not recommend travel restrictions or specific health measures for the travelers? Also, screening at entry points was thought to offer a limited benefit while using up a lot of resources.

On the 27th of January 2020, WHO issued an updated report which confirmed human to human transmission of the disease? Measures were aimed at reducing the risk of importation and exportation of the disease without non-essential restrictions. General health measures to follow by travelers and country health authorities were the same as that of the earlier report. Measures on entry and exit point screening were also given in the report.

On the 30th of January 2020, COVID-19 was declared a public health emergency of international concern (PHEIC) by the WHO. Countries were advised to be prepared for containment, screening, isolation, diagnosis, case management, contact tracing, and identification. Specific measures were issued related to repatriation and quarantine of travelers.

On the 4th of February 2020, CDC also issued a Level 3 warning to avoid non-essential travel to China. Transportation within and out of the affected province of China were also affected. The US Department of State also issued a Level 4 advisory asking people not to travel to China due to the coronavirus outbreak.

If someone must travel to China, they are to follow the preventive guidelines as stated earlier. Cancellation or postponement of travel to Hong Kong was not recommended by CDC. Travelers to Hong Kong are encouraged to practice the usual precautions.

Health Professionals

Specific guidelines were issued in order to guide healthcare facilities and health professionals on infection prevention and control measures in the management of suspected and confirmed cases of 2019-nCoV infection.

As the spectrum of disease is largely unknown, a criteria was devised to evaluate a patient. Healthcare providers are to obtain detailed information on the travel history of patients being evaluated for fever and acute respiratory illness.

Healthcare providers stand at great risk of acquiring the

infection because of the frequent contact with infected patients. Healthcare providers should adhere to infection control and prevention strategies to protect themselves from acquiring the infection. It includes the appropriate use of engineering, administrative controls, and personal protective equipment (PPE). Guidance about the appropriate use of personal protective equipment has been issued by the CDC.

Hand hygiene should be maintained using alcohol-based hand sanitizer before and after every patient contact, or contact with materials that could be potentially infectious, as well as before putting on and taking off protective equipment, gloves inclusive. Routine cleaning and disinfection procedures should be performed. Management of laundry, food service utensils and medical waste should also be performed per guidelines. A health care provider who has an unprotected exposure to a confirmed or possible case 2019-nCoV patient should quickly contact their supervisor or occupational health officer. If a health professional starts having symptoms consistent with COV 19 infection, they should not report to work but instead, should contact their occupational health services.

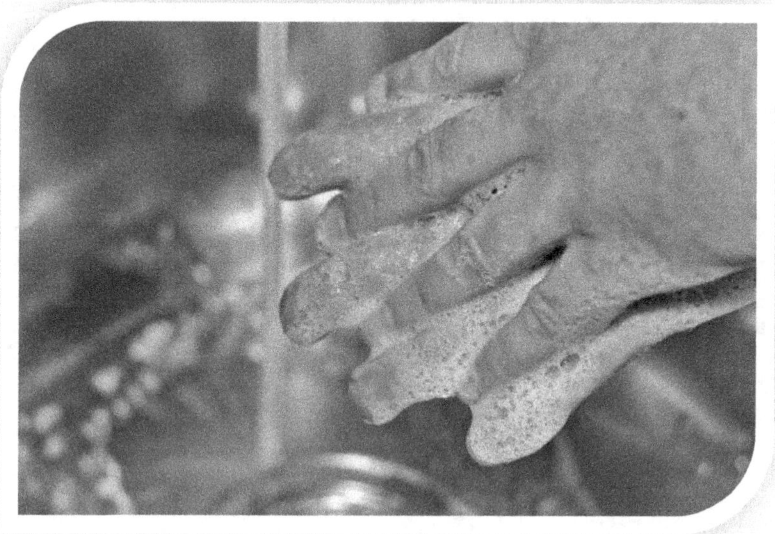

Business

Guidelines for employers to use:

Encouraging sick employees to stay home. Employees should notify their seniors and stay home if they are sick. Flexible policies that allow employees to remain home to care for ill family members should be encouraged.

Sick employees should be kept away from others and wear a facemask. They should cover their faces while coughing and sneezing.

Encouragement of hygienic practices like hand washing in offices.

Persons infected With Coronavirus

If a person was in China in the preceeding 14 days and feels sick with fever, cough, or difficulty in breathing, they should:

Consult a medical doctor – They should call ahead before they go to a doctor's office or emergency room and should reveal all relevant information.

Not come in contact with other people.

Wash the hand with water together with soap immediately after coughing, sneezing or blowing the nose. If soap and water are not available, sanitizer can be used. If hands are visibly soiled, washing them with soap is always preferred.

Clean and disinfect contact surfaces.

If a person falls ill, they should:

- *Stay at home and restrict movements except to seek medical care.*
- *Avoid the use of public transportation.*
- *Isolate themselves. Contact with other people and animals during illness should be very minimal.*

- *Inform the doctor before visiting so that steps may be taken to prevent other people from getting exposed.*

- *Wear a facemask when they come in contact with other people.*

- *Cover their mouth and nose during coughing or sneezing.*

- *Refrain from sharing household personal items with other people*

- *Practice handwashing with water and soap.*

- *Avoid touching the eyes, mouth and nose with dirty hands.*

- *Disinfect the touched surfaces and maintain a clean environment.*

- *Monitor their symptoms and seek medical care if symptoms get worse.*

MYTHS AND FACTS

There has been misinformation and hoaxes accompanying the rapid spread of the Wuhan coronavirus (also known as 2019-nCoV). Some of the hoaxes include how to treat it, it's spread and false claims about its source. It is unarguable that this is a dangerous development.

In this branch, you will discover these myths and why they are wrong.

Myth 1: Antibiotics Are an Effective Remedy

Antibiotics do not work against viruses; it works against bacteria. 2019-nCoV is a virus. Persons with bacterial co-infection are usually given antibiotics.

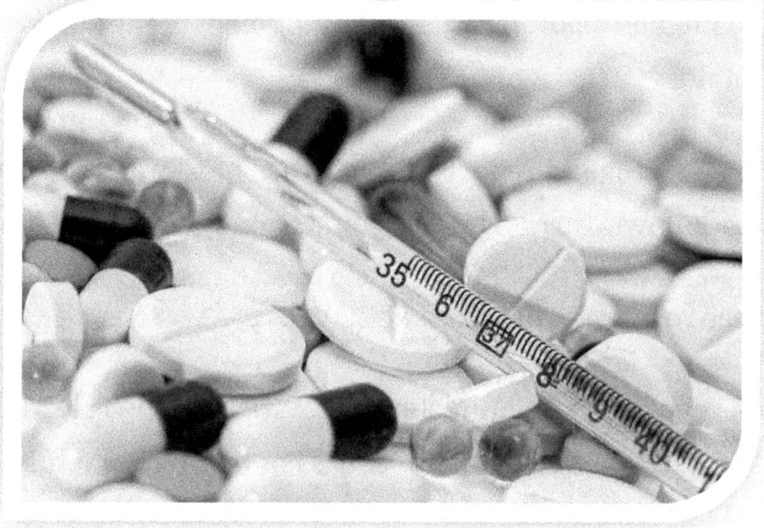

Myth 2: This Virus Only Affects Old People

Anyone regardless of age can be infected by this virus. The only difference is that people, especially old people are more susceptible to the virus's infection because they have pre-existing medical conditions like heart disease, diabetes, and asthma.

Are there any specific medicines to forestall or treat the new coronavirus?

To date, there's no specific medicine recommended to forestall or treat the new coronavirus (2019-nCoV).

FACT CHECK! COVID-19 Timeline

The Timeline below tracks the development of the outbreak as it unfolds.

Feb. 26 — Algeria reports its first case of COVID-19 — an Italian adult, who arrived in the country on Feb. 17.

Greece reports its first case of COVID-19.

Iran's deputy health minister, Iraj Harirchi, who is leading the nation's COVID-19 task force, has contracted the virus.

Cases in China are falling, according to Dr. Bruce Aylward, who led the external experts on a mission in China for the past two weeks — from an average of 2,500 cases two weeks ago to 400 cases today. But he warned against complacency.

Kuwait, Bahrain, Afghanistan, Iraq, and Oman report first cases of COVID-19.

Feb. 23 — South Korean President Moon Jae-in announces the highest level of alert after the country surpasses 340 cases of COVID-19, the majority of which were discovered in the past few days.

In a speech at the Munich Security Conference, WHO Director-General Tedros Adhanom Ghebreyesus called for an increase in funding to the response. "We're concerned by the lack of urgency in funding the response from the international community," he said.

Egypt reports its first case of COVID-19. This is the first case confirmed on the African continent and the first new country to see a case since Feb. 4.

There could be information in a matter of weeks about the impact of drugs currently in trial to treat the virus, according to WHOM.

WHO says 17 countries in Africa now have the capacity to test for COVID-19. This is a clarification from Feb. 7, when WHO had said 28 countries in Africa have the capacity.

A total of 175 people test positive for COVID-19 on the Diamond Princess Cruise ship, which is quarantined in Japan.

A United Nations Crisis Management Team is activated, led by Dr. Michael Ryan, executive director at WHO's Health Emergencies Programmed.

WHO says a vaccine could be available in an estimated 18 months.

168 labs around the world now have the capacity to diagnose the virus.

Feb. 9 — the death toll of victims of the 2019-nCoV is now

over 800, surpassing the death toll of the SARS epidemic in 2002 and 2003, which killed 773 people.

Get development's most important headlines in your inbox every day.

Four main possible future evolutions and scenarios

1. The spread of the virus gets under control thanks to public health authorities interventions. This is what happened with the SARS. In this way affected people immune systems can fight the virus without it spreading to anyone new. In the unfortunate cases, the virus will kill the patient, and it goes down with them.

2. A pandemic develops proximate, China's aggressive actions stop the virus but as cases decrease and restriction ease new infections occur outside China afterwards

3. Coronavirus becomes another common virus, it becomes a seasonal disease, the coronavirus becomes a regular part of cold and flu season.

4. Future will be a combination of scenarios 1 to 5.

What can the economic impacts be

The trade war between United States and China, where

tariffs were on specific imported goods, caused a significant slowdown in manufacturing in 2019. The coronavirus is both manufacturing hurting both manufacturing and service industries. Tourism could be one of the main sector impacted. As of February 2020 IATA (International Air Transport Association) have revised their forecast as results of the coronavirus COVID-19

- IATA forecast for air travel demand growth in 2020 initially estimated at 4.1% has been revised to a contraction of 0.6% (based on SARS case)

- Cost for airlines estimated at around 29 billion dollar in revenues (overall about -5%/-6% vs beginning of the year 2020 estimate)

- Lower fuel costs could however help margins offsetting some of the lost revenue

- Delay in planned investments from Airlines may occur across different areas IT included

Impacts in service industries are particularly relevant for the United States, where service industries are the majority of the economic activity.

In addition while tariffs add challenges for global commerce, that has different implications than shutting down entirely. With trade tariff enterprises have other options e.g. sourcing goods from elsewhere or simply paying more for them.

In case of a production crisis/shut down, governmental and central banks actions and policies to stimulate demand may have very limited effects if there is a strong issue on the offer side. Fed and other central banks may take action to try to shield the world economy from those shocks. However monetary policy or fiscal policy mainly acts on the demand side. E.g. lower interest rates will not heal a sick person.

Some estimates as of February 2020 show the following

- China's economic growth set to slow down to 4.5% in the first quarter of 2020 – the slowest growth since the 2007 financial crisis, according to a Reuters poll of economists

- Global oil demand had had a strong impact has declared by the International Energy Agency

- Factory shutdowns are decreasing the inflow of products and parts from China, impacting companies around the world.

The most likely scenario that is floating around is:

- A SARS similar impact, temporary slowdown, outbreak is contained and stopped within China and other few areas where it has reached

- Outbreak is not contained, impact are on the overall global economy. This context could however drive more insourcing, i.e. put production where customer actually is, in order to minimize occasions for contagion. E.g. American Companies increasing production capacity in the US.

What can companies do?

Companies should consider to think about plans in order be ready in case a crisis hits.

The health of employees is essential as people are a critical resource. It may be needed to rethink work practices. This obviously depends on the job requirements.

Emergency operations center should exist at the corporate, business unit but also plant level. With clear action plans for communication and coordination, roles, protocols for decision making. Business should also identify criticalities and dependencies in the supply chain. Companies around the world have been operating under the assumption that materials flow without issues globally. Therefore companies have been able to source, produce, and distribute products at the lowest-cost locations around the world. However trade wars (US/China), Brexit, and now the coronavirus have challenged the assumption. The coronavirus shows the exposures generated by having the majority of the production deployments in the same one area. Companies need to think differently in terms of how to configure their supply chains. One option is to have backup capacity for supply, production, and distribution outages. So spreading the risk of a disruption across two sources in two very different locations. Another option could be to have production deployed locally e.g. in each of the major markets.

These options spread the risk, therefore supporting better responses to situation of crises and business continuity. Also transportation costs may be lower. However as productions is more dispersed, there may be lower economies of scale, higher capital costs, higher administrative, quality monitoring and finally higher unit costs.

Common conspiracy theories floating around

Although none of the below backed up by facts some sites have reported some conspiracies theories:

- American bio-weapon, theory supposedly pushed by Russia, was the bio-weapon was intended to slow down China's economic development.

- Chinese leaked biological weapon, fed by the fact that Wuhan is home to one of China's top-level bio-research facilities, the Wuhan Institute of Virology

- Big plot by pharmaceutical companies to get rich.

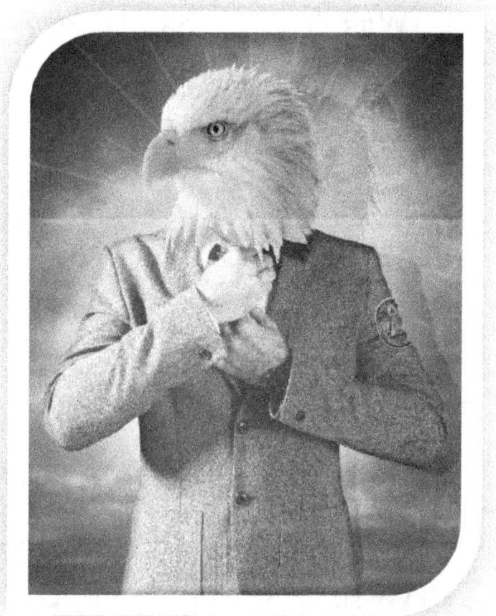

HOW TO PROTECT YOURSELF FROM ILLNESS

Important Steps to Take to Keep from Getting Sick

1. *Wash your hands regularly*

Wash your hands every couple hours, whether you remember touching something suspect or not. If you have touched something that is suspect, wash your hands immediately.

2. *Moisturize*

Moisturizing your skin helps to keep it strong and malleable. Your skin is your first and greatest defense from infection and illness, so keeping it from getting cracked and dry will help you to fight off illnesses.

3. *Wash your hands after handling money*

Even if you only slipped your credit card or debit card through the little reader, rub your hands with sanitizer or wash your hands thoroughly. Money is one of the primary means for the conveyance of illness from one person to another, even more so than toilet seats.

4. *Sanitize your phone frequently*

If you are like most of the general population today, you touch your phone on a nearly constant basis. Doing so means that any of the germs you pick up from any other things or places you touch are put on the phone, then subsequently spread around, no matter how frequently you wash your hands. Using a disinfectant wipe a couple times throughout the day (particularly if you bring your phone into the bathroom and set it down) should help to get the job done with no problem.

5. *Don't touch your face*

Your face is sensitive and can absorb germs. Aside from this, you can touch your nose, mouth, and eyes, which allow you to pick up some of your own germs and spread them all over. Keeping your hands away from your face can help keep the spread of sickness down from others to you and vice versa.

6. *Refrain from picking your nose*

This one might seem obvious, but it's just a force of habit for some people. This is one of the fastest ways to spread illness. By picking your nose and touching things around you, you leave others to pick up those germs proximate on. Not to mention the fact that, if you have germs on your finger when you put it in your nose, you're putting those germs into your sinuses.

7. *Sanitize after blowing your nose*

If you blow your nose, use a little bit of hand sanitizer to kill any germs and make sure to put your tissue in a bag that you can close up at the end of the day. This can help you to keep from spreading germs around the home or workplace.

8. *Vampire cough*

If you happen to have a tickle in your throat, use the crook of your elbow to obscure your mouth while you cough to clear it. This keeps the spread of germs from being quite so simple and it will keep you from coughing on anyone.

9. *Sanitize or disinfect shared surfaces*

If there are spaces that are shared with you and another person, just give them a quick wipe-down with a disinfectant wipe or a little spritz of disinfectant cleaner to make sure that everything is left fresh and clean.

10. Prepare your own food

Going out to eat while there is a widespread illness is a big role of the dice. Many people who work in foodservice can't afford to take sick leave and are pressured by management to work in spite of symptoms, as a way to combat chronic understaffing. As a means of avoiding this, you can and should prepare your own food and eat at home to keep yourself healthy in the middle of an outbreak.

11. Avoid salad bars

Salad bars and buffet-style restaurants have sneeze guards over the food, but those foods are ultimately left in the open air for a good deal of time. If someone didn't wash their hands before handling the spoon or tongs on the buffet, they have spread their germs to that entire dish.

12. Don't pick at your teeth or put your fingers in your mouth

Putting your fingers into your mouth puts your germs out into the area as well as putting any germs you picked up, right into your mouth. If you have something your teeth, go to the bathroom and wash your hands before and after picking at it. It is optimal to also use a flosser in addition to this hand-washing precaution.

How to Properly Wash Your Hands

For many who have never worked in food service or in the medical field, the proper method for hand washing tends to get a little bit overlooked. For many people, washing your hands simply means putting a little bit of soap on the hands and then rinsing it off.

Antibacterial soap typically needs about 20 seconds to fully cleanse an area on which it's being used. This means that the couple of seconds that you run your hand under the tap with a little blob of soap on your hands does after to nothing to fight off infection, germs, bacteria, or illness.

The proper method for washing your hands is as follows:

1. Wet your hands with warm water and turn off the tap.

2. Apply soap to your hands in a generous, but not overabundant amount.

3. Rub the soap into your hands to create bubbles, making sure to rub the soap in between your fingers, onto the back of your hands, and up your wrists. Continue this for 20 seconds.

4. Rinse your hands under the warm water to rid your hands of bubbles.

5. Pat or wipe your hands dry on a clean towel.

This is the proper method for washing your hands, no matter what type of soap you're using and to make sure that you're using this method each and every time you wash your hands will ensure that you're not retaining extra germs and you won't be spreading them around by using your hands.

What Types of Masks Work Against Viruses?

If you're looking to fight off a virus, infection, disease, or illness by improving the quality of the air you're breathing, you will want a mask that is marked "disposable respirator." You will commonly see this type of mask marked as N95 or P2. Make sure that the packaging for the mask you buy specifically states that it will prevent the conveyance or communication of illnesses.

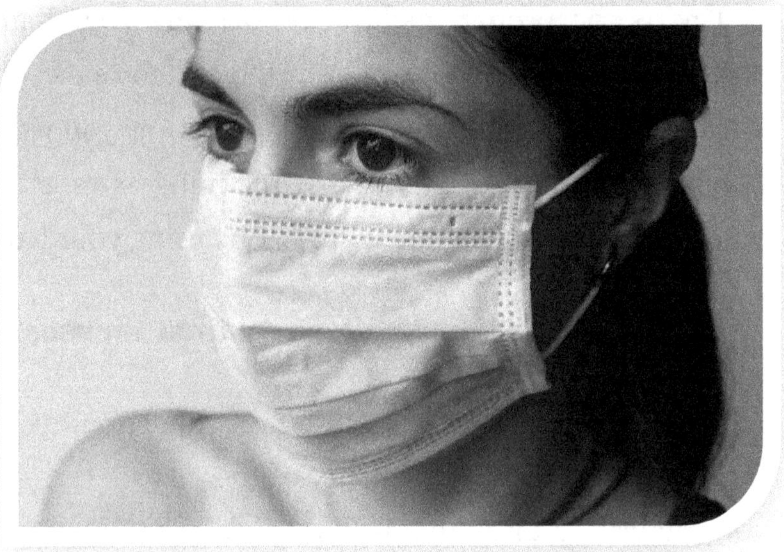

Taking this little extra step to make sure that you're not breathing in the particulates from anyone's nose, mouth, etc., can help you to keep yourself safe from those illnesses while you're out and about running errands or doing the things you need to do in public.

If you're trying to keep your respiratory health safeguarded, you must make sure that you have the right masks for the situation you find yourself in.

- For Smoke: particulate respirators, N95, P100, and NIOSH masks can help to protect your lungs from the harsh smoke in a fire.

- For Pollution: N95 masks are best for air pollution.

- For Dust: N95 or R95 masks can help to keep dust and oily particulates from getting into your lungs.

- For Contagion: DFM, N95, and P2 masks are the best to keep your lungs safe from harmful contagions, mists, fumes, and dust. You can also look for something labeled "disposable respirator."

Types of Disinfectants

When you're trying to keep yourself and your spaces clear of illnesses and germs, you want to make sure that you're using the right material for the job.

- Hand Sanitizer: This is best for use in a pinch. It's great to use right after handling money at the grocery store, right after blowing your nose, or when you're going into a meeting and need to shake some hands with people. Washing your hands is always the best possible option for keeping your hands clean, but hand sanitizer is a great stop-gap.

- Spray disinfectant: These are the things like Lysol™ that can be used to cling to and neutralize the bacteria or particulates in the air that might be cause for concern, and they also have products that you can put directly onto surfaces to clean them.

- Bleach: This is a very harsh disinfectant, but it will kill just about anything it touches in terms of germs. If you have items that are made of plastic or that won't be damaged by chlorine, you can soak them in a solution of bleach and water to completely sanitize them.

- Hydrogen Peroxide: This is great to use to clear away any bacteria that might be around a minor cut, scrape, or bruise. It's best to use this right after the moment of injury to see to it that no infection or contamination occurs.

Herbal Remedies for Immune Support

Herbal remedies are a very popular solution to common illnesses like the cold and the flu. These can be very soothing and helpful, as well as easy on the body. Some harsher medicines can leave you with certain side-effects and, if the illness is dire enough, they may be a necessary evil.

If you prefer to use herbal remedies such as rose hips, Echinacea, and some homeopathic remedies as well, that is fine to do as long as it doesn't conflict with or hinder the doctor's orders. If your doctor has prescribed something to you and is telling you that simple home remedies won't do the trick to get you on the path to wellness, you owe it to yourself and to everyone around you to listen to that advice.

By all means, take your vitamins, drink your tea, eat your soup, and use all the natural remedies that helped you to cope with illness in the past. Just don't take things that will cancel out your current medical treatment for the illness you have, and follow your doctor's instructions to the letter. This is the best, fastest, and most ideal route to getting better as quickly as possible.

Proper Medical Care

There is nothing wrong with making sure that you're getting the best possible medical care for your conditions or illnesses. If you feel like your doctor may have made an error in your medical treatment, seek a second opinion from other trusted professionals in the field. If you have reason to believe that the advice of a non-medical person may be more correct than that of a licensed professional, get that advice checked thoroughly before following it.

Your life is precious, so make sure that you're trusting the best possible sources for information on how to recover from an illness or how to properly treat one. Take the medications that are prescribed to you if you aren't allergic to them and do your best to follow the medical advice that you've been given by the trained, licensed professionals in charge of your care.

How to Keep Yourself Well During Treatment

1. Keep Your Nutrition on Track

If you're anything like me, being at home all day can cause you to want to snack a lot. If you're going to be stuck in the house for a long time, you're going to want to keep your food rationed out properly to make sure that it lasts, and you're going to want to make sure that the foods you're eating contribute to good, proper nutrition. When your body is able to work off of the right kinds of fuel, it is much more ready to fight off the things that are attacking its internal systems.

This means that you'll want to make sure that you're getting plenty of protein, the right kinds and amounts of carbs, a good amount of fiber, fresh fruits and vegetables, foods that are rich in vitamins and minerals, and plenty of water. These are things that you should be getting on a daily basis and, if you aren't typically seeing yourself eat like this, then there's no time like the present!

Getting onto a better, healthier regimen of eating when you get sick can give your system the boost it needs to fight off the nasty virus it's working against and it can help you to feel a lot less run-down while you're trying to recover. Consider the kind of healthier foods you would like to eat while you're stuck at home and think of some creative ways to make them into dishes that you like, which fill you up, and which give your body the right amounts of the right kinds of fuel.

This doesn't have to be a drastic change and you don't have to switch over to anything like an all-raw vegan diet or anything. It's just best to make sure that the types of foods you're putting in your body are healthy, diverse, and contain all the good stuff your body needs to thrive.

2. Get Plenty of Rest

When you're sick with a cold, the flu, or anything worse, it's a great idea to make sure that you're getting all the rest you possibly can. If your cough and shortness of breath makes it hard for you to get proper rest when you're lying down flat, prop yourself up with pillows to keep you sitting up or to keep you on your side.

For many people, falling asleep while they're sick is simply involuntary. Watching television or doing something that doesn't require that the mind be too engaged will allow them to just drift off to sleep for as long as their body needs them to do so. Sleeping through the night can be hard while you're sick, but speak with your doctor about the possibility of using a sleep aid or a cough syrup with drowsy effects to help you to get the very most sleep you possibly can.

When your body is asleep, a lot less of its energy is going to things like walking around, paying attention, and operating at higher levels. When you're asleep, everything slows down and your body is given the chance to relax a bit and switch all the energy over to the immune processes that are fighting to keep you healthy.

3. Drink Plenty of Fluids

Drinking enough fluids when you're sick can be tricky since you're sleeping so much. Try to fit in some water and even some electrolytes whenever you possibly can. If you can find some electrolyte solution and add it to your water, you will find that it helps your cells to be able to absorb more of what you're drinking and can make it more beneficial to the body.

It can be hard to know what enough water is for a person who is sick and trying to recover from it. For the average person, half a gallon is the daily recommended intake. For someone who is sick, it should be about half again as much. If you are someone who finds that they are constantly running to and from the bathroom when they drink this amount of water, I have a little analogy and a tip for you.

Have you ever tried to pour a whole cup of water into a thirsty plant, only to see it just kind overflow out of the sides before it can soak in? With that same plant, if you were to pour a little bit at a time, the plant would drink it all up and within just a couple of days, you would see more bright greenery on that little plant!

It has been found that your body can absorb up to eight ounces of fluid within a 15-minute span. This means that if you have a 32-ounce cup of water in front of you, you should take about an hour to finish it. Doing so will allow your body to soak in and use all the water that you're giving to it, and it will also make it much easier to get that much water into your system overall!

4. Avoid Sugars

Sugary foods and drinks can drastically dehydrate your body. Doing this when you're sick can set you back quite a ways when you're trying to recover and get better. Your body has to work hard to break down those sugars that you put into your body, and it can cause your blood sugar to spike. When this happens, your body has a little bit more work to do than it would if you ate a cucumber of a piece of chicken instead.

While you're trying to let your body heal from this illness and while you're trying to give your immune system all the power it could possibly need to fight off the illness, you will want to cut back on things like sugary drinks, candy, ice cream, and foods with low nutritional value and high amounts of filler or sugar.

Doing so might be the last thing you're thinking about doing when you're trying to fight off an illness that is serious, and that is a notion that I understand very well. I simply leave you with this information about possible avenues that you can take as a way to help your body to recover faster and in greater strides.

5. Keep Yourself Busy

Don't allow yourself to get so bored that you can't stand being home anymore! Pick up little creative projects, projects that you've been meaning to get around to, things you've always wanted to try but never had time, games you've wanted to play, reading pamphlet that you want to read, and anything else you can think of.

Keeping your mind engaged, keeping your brain working, and keeping yourself feeling like you've got lots of things to do and work on will keep you from feeling too isolated. Fighting the feeling of isolation can be just as much a struggle as fighting the illness itself, so don't let it take a back seat when you're making arrangements for your treatment and your quarantine.

WHAT TO DO DURING A QUARANTINE

If you have been ordered to stay at home to prevent the spread of an illness, you want to make sure that you have all the things you could possibly need to get you through that quarantine. You will want to make sure that you have enough food, entertainment, medical supplies, first aid, and anything else that you could possibly need over that two-week span.

If you are sick, you might need tissues, prescription medicine, soup, lip balm, a thermometer, and other things that help you to feel comforted and well while you're trying to get better. If you are helping someone in your home, that is sick, you might need to make sure that you have phamplet or puzzles to keep yourself busy during the day.

A good basic list of things to keep in the house can be found in Episode Three, but I have modified the list specifically for quarantine and listed it here:

Water. You need to drink plenty of fluids when you're sick,

so make sure that you have enough for about ¾ of a gallon per person, per day for the duration of your quarantine.

Food. If you are quarantined, you may need to procure enough food to last you for two weeks. Consider grocery delivery to your home if you need to stock up as soon as you are quarantined and have the delivery person leave the groceries on the doorstep, only opening the door once they have gone away. This will help to prevent the spread of illness.

A first aid kit with all the bells and whistles. Many of the first aid kits that are available for purchase online come with things that you can use for symptom suppression as well as things to treat wounds. It's best to have one of these on hand when you're quarantined, just in case of anything that might happen.

Face masks to help you to breathe contaminated air. Make sure that you have the right masks for the situation you find yourself in. DFM, N95, and P2 masks are the best to keep your lungs safe from harmful contagions, mists, fumes, and dust. You can also look for something labeled "disposable respirator."

Sanitary products. If the person or people who are going to be quarantined are menstruating or could be during the time of the quarantine, it's best to stock up and make sure that you have any menstrual cups, pads, tampons, pant liners, wipes, or whatever other products might be needed. As a side note to this, if there are any foods that help to cope with cramping or symptoms of the period, you will want to stock up on those as well.

Entertainment. Do not underestimate how easy it is to go completely stir-crazy when staying in the house for two full weeks, especially if you're in there with other people. You want to make sure that you have games to play, television to watch, phamplet to read, activities to do with one another, as well as on your own, and you want to make sure that there is always something to keep your attention.

Don't Travel

This one might seem really obvious to you, but it has to be said. If you are diagnosed with the illness, you should not travel anywhere. This does, unfortunately, apply if you are abroad when you are diagnosed. You need to find somewhere local to where you were diagnosed to stay until it's fully treated.

Traveling through areas that have not yet been exposed to the illness opens them up to new, more wide-spread cases. It is better to have 1,000 infected people all in one city than it is to have 500 infected people all across the globe. Those 500 people could come into contact with hundreds, if not thousands of people within the incubation period and could infect countless other people, making it imperative that you stay right where you are following diagnosis and pending treatment.

Wear Masks When Accepting Deliveries

It's best to avoid getting deliveries at all if you're in the middle of treatment for COVID-19, but if you find that you are out of something you desperately need, there may not be an alternative. If it's possible, the best option would be for the delivery person to drop the products at the door and leave before you open it. If this isn't something they can do or if they need you to sign a receipt, be sure to very, very thoroughly wash and sanitize your hands, wear a mask when you open the door, and use a spray disinfectant to treat the air around you when you open the door.

This might seem like overkill, but delivery people deal with lots of stop every single day. That could be at least a hundred more people exposed in one week after delivering to your home.

Don't Break Your Quarantine, Even if You Feel Better

As mentioned earlier, it is quite possible to still be carrying COVID-19 after your symptoms have subsided. If your doctor has advised that you keep yourself at home and away from others for a specific period of time, you should keep to that limit in spite of how you feel.

For other illnesses that affect these parts of the body, it's possible to feel better, branch out and do more in your day, only to find that you overdid it and suddenly your symptoms are back in full swing. What does that tell you? It says that the illness has not yet left your body, but that your immune system was just really working hard that day and starting to win the battle. Go outdoors, exert yourself just a little too much and your symptoms are back. In any case, you're exposing anyone around you to COVID-19 and it's just not safe.

When it comes to quarantines, the entire philosophy is based on the notion that it's better to be safe than it is to be sorry! For people with compromised immune systems and even for some who aren't compromised, coronavirus can be fatal. There just isn't anything you can do to apologize enough for spreading that kind of illness by breaking your quarantine, so it's best to just stay put.

No Visitors

The principle behind this is just the same as it is with breaking the quarantine and with getting deliveries. Having company can be really, really tempting if you've been alone in your quarantine for two weeks, but you can get through it. You can voice chat with people, call them on the phone, play video games online, video call, and anything that would allow you to connect with family that are not near you. Doing this is a great way to keep yourself from feeling too isolated while you're being cut off from the rest of the world.

Do your best to fight the temptation to have visitors in your home during your quarantine. In fact, you should do your best to keep visitors from coming to your home until you've had the chance to properly sanitize everything once the illness has passed. Wash all the pillows, pillowcases, sheets, blankets, and clothing. Sanitize all the surfaces, dust, vacuum, and get brand new toothbrushes. You don't want any possibility of the virus or germs to be lurking around in your home to latch onto anyone who comes to visit you.

Don't Share Germs, No Matter What

If you and someone else happen to be quarantined together

and you are both affected by COVID-19, it is still not a good idea to share cups, dishes, or food. The transference of contaminants from one patient to another is still a concern for the doctors who are working to treat the illness and who are trying to find the best avenues for treating and curing the illness.

Because people are walking incubators, the virus could behave differently once it's inside you than it might inside the other person. Because that person is working to fight off the illness when a new mutation of it enters their body, they might be unprepared to fight it off, causing more problems for you, that person, their doctor, or anyone else who happens to be involved in the quarantine or treatment.

Disinfect Surfaces Regularly

While you're stuck in quarantine, it's a good practice to make sure that you're routinely disinfecting surfaces and cleaning up any messes that collect in the house. Studies show that a cleaner, more orderly environment is more conducive to faster healing from illnesses and injuries. It can also be helpful to give yourself maintenance tasks around the home in order to keep yourself busy for a portion of each day.

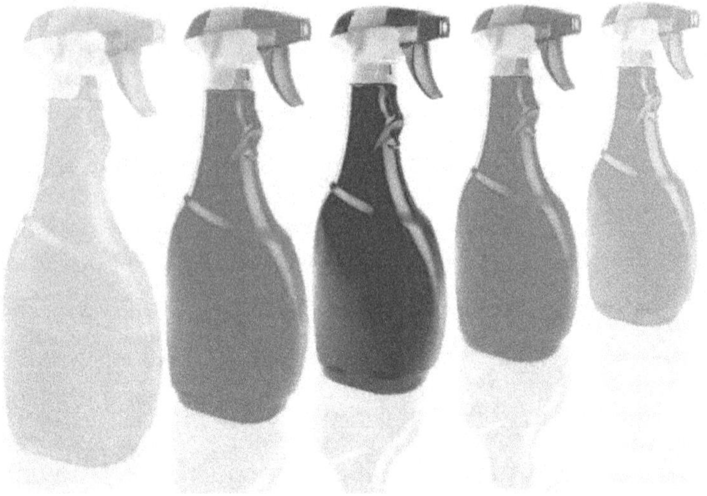

You can also consider taking on a small cleaning or organizing project to take yourself from room to room to clean things up as you're spending time in the house. Make sure you don't push yourself too hard and overdo it, but giving yourself something to focus on and something to work toward can help you to feel better faster, and it can help you to occupy a lot of time that might otherwise be filled with boredom and wishing that you weren't still stuck in that one space.

Call for Medical Assistance When Needed

When you are sent into quarantine by your doctor, it's typical for them to give you a particular protocol to follow in the event that you need medical assistance. In many cases, it won't be fine for you to just hop in the car and drive down to the doctor's office if something is wrong.

You will likely need to call your doctor, explain the nature of the problem that led you to call and arrange for a professional medical transport to your doctor or to a medical facility that is equipped to help you.

When you're quarantined, you have to plan every move you make with the help of your doctor to make sure that you're not going to step on any regulations, that you're not going to cause any problems, and that you're not going to make yourself any sicker. With the professional medical advice given to you by your doctor, you have the best possible chance to getting through your illness with as little hassle as possible.

How to Handle Quarantine with One Sick Family Member

It is an unfortunate possibility for one member of your family to become sick and to need to be quarantined in the home with the rest of the family. In many cases where there isn't overcrowding in the hospitals, such cases are kept in the hospital. In many cases as well, the patient can be given a choice depending on the severity of the illness. This may or may not be an option that the doctor will consider or allow, but just in case, it's best to have all the information about how you can keep yourself and your family safe, happy, and healthy throughout the quarantine.

Wear a Mask when Helping the Patient

If the patient, your family member, is staying in your home, it's a great idea to try to limit their activity to one part of the house so everyone else can interact without the fear of infection. If you decide this is the best possible option, you should wear a mask while you're in that room to help them with food, getting dressed, or whatever other help the person may require.

In some cases, as when the patient is a child, they might need more contact and more closeness than someone who is more independent might. It's imperative that you make sure you are as protected during these interactions as possible. Rubber gloves may be a good idea to help keep your hands from coming into contact with infectious materials. Speak with your doctor about what other measures you can take to ensure that you're safe while providing support and comfort for your affected family member.

Putting ourselves at risk in order to accommodate or help a family member—particularly our children—is something that appeals to many of us and it might seem like the right idea at the time to stay with your child in spite of the risk. With an illness such as this one, it is best to keep yourself safe and to avoid contracting the illness at all costs. You can provide the best possible care for your child when you are feeling your best.

Quarantine the Patient in Their Room

Keeping the patient—your family member—in their room while they recover is the best possible option you and the rest of your family have for keeping that sickness at bay. Make sure that the person has access to all the things they could need in order to keep themselves occupied and entertained while they're stuck in there, but it's best not to spend too much time in the room with them.

With all the avenues for personal entertainment, there is a wealth of options available to keep someone busy while they're stuck in their room. Video games, pamphlet , movies, TV shows, puzzles, mobile games, audio, crafts, crochet, knitting, macramé, building blocks, toys, model building, magazines, music, coloring, drawing, and so much more.

If your family member is having a hard time choosing something they think they would like to do, help them to narrow it down and make a coin flip or dice rolling randomizer to help them choose something. Pick six things you feel like doing, assign each one a unique number from one to six, roll the die and bingo! There's the first task for you to do.

Being creative is the best possible way to keep yourself from feeling too isolated during a quarantine, so get to thinking! Talk with your family member about the types of things they like to do in order to pass the time when they're by themselves and help them to get what they need in order to get it done!

Disinfect All Surfaces in the House

I know I sound like a broken record on this particular point, but it's even more important if you have one sick person in the house and you're trying to keep everyone else from getting the illness. Using a disinfectant solution of some kind, make sure to wipe down all the surfaces in your house at least once a day. Bathroom counter, kitchen counters, the top of the island in the kitchen if you have one, the coffee table, the end tables, and for good measure, you may as well get all the doorknobs while you're at it.

If you know of things that are being handled a lot in the house like remotes, video game controllers and cell phones, go ahead and sanitize those as well. Doing so will help to keep everyone's hands a little bit cleaner. Everyone should also be committed to washing their hands regularly, keeping their hands away from their noses, mouths, ears, and faces, and making sure that they're keeping things clean if they have touched body fluids like mucus, tears, or saliva.

Keep Conflicts to a Minimum and Resolve them Quickly

With families, there will always be the occasional spat or argument to defuse. When you and your family are kept in close quarters for a long period of time, it can cause those things to come up a little more frequently. When those things do come up, it's important to be able to help everyone to reach an agreement and settle those arguments quickly. Letting them continue or ramp up in intensity will only serve to sour the mood in the house and to make life a little bit harder for everyone to cope with.

If you are able to resolve conflicts, then you should absolutely do so. If a resolution simply doesn't seem possible, then the arguing parties should make it a point to separate themselves from one another to give the rest of the family peace. Conflict resolution can be difficult and it's not ideal for the entire family to get involved over every single dispute.

That being said, there are cases in which a little bit of mediation and intervention can help to calm things down, put things in perspective, and to help all involved parties to feel as though they've been heard. Sometimes, a proper acknowledgment is all it takes for two people to admit to one another that the argument was more intense than it needed to be and that they can behave amicably from that point forward.

If you are unclear on how to resolve and calm down conflicts, take a look into some conflict resolution tools online to help you to get an edge on it. Sometimes, it doesn't even need to be the other person in the argument acknowledging someone and their point of view to cool things down. If you can tell someone, "I see what you're saying and I get why you feel that way," it can really help them to come around and to stop seeing the situation as being quite so adversarial.

Play Games to Keep Everyone Occupied

Games are a great way to keep the whole family engaged, occupied, happy, and entertained. It gets people talking, it helps people to work together, it stimulates the mind, and it helps to pass the time much more easily. I would recommend against games that inspire people to get too competitive or upset in the process, but for the most part, you will find that board games are a great way to go.

If you are a family that likes to play video games or do crafts together as well, then you should absolutely make the necessary provisions to be able to do that during the time of your quarantine.

IMPORTANT TERMS TO KNOW

1. ENDEMIC

Adjective. (Of a condition or of a disease) prevalent or found regularly among a particular population, group or area.

When a disease is endemic, it means that it's commonplace amongst certain people, certain places, and in certain conditions. One would say that the common cold is endemic in the wintertime. It's almost like you can expect people to come down with this particular illness when it's this time of year or when certain conditions are present.

"The bends are endemic amongst deep-sea divers and diving enthusiasts."

As of right now, coronavirus cannot be considered endemic. It is not nearly widespread enough for this and it's not as common as the news reports and viral media may have us believe. While it is a prevalent problem, it is far from reaching the endemic status those organizations such as the CDC or WHO would have to give it.

An illness that has become endemic are the ones that can predictably occur within a certain group, population, or in areas where specific conditions are typically present. One of the more well-known endemic illnesses in the United States is chicken pox. Most children who are young and in school, typically of about eight years of age or below, can be expected to contract and display symptoms of chicken pox. The disease is nearly always present in a given community, but in fairly low frequency.

In short, endemic illnesses and diseases are the ones that can be trusted to occur semi-frequently but are not a great cause for concern as we have figured out treatment for them and are quick to administer it when the time comes for us to do so. If your doctor has treatment or prevention options for such illnesses, such as vaccines and courses of medicinal treatment, it is best to follow their professional medical advice for the best possible results.

Noun. A prevalent spread of an infectious disease or illness within a community (large or small), striking many people and causing illness all at once.

2. EPIDEMIC

Adjective. Having the nature or scope of an illness that is an epidemic.

Epidemic is probably the most commonly used word with the "-demic" suffix. This is the one that indicates a sudden, severe, and widespread of active cases of illness within a specific community or area. Epidemics can be on a small scale, like a school having several widespread cases throughout the different classrooms and grades.

The CDC says that an epidemic can occur when there are an adequate number of susceptible hosts and an adequate number of people carrying the illness in question are in a specific area. This allows the illness to branch out from the agent to those susceptible hosts and to take hold there. From there, the spread can continue in just the same way, causing a rash of cases in a short period of time, typically right inside the incubation period.

Being a susceptible host means that your immune system is either compromised or simply unacquainted with the illness enough to fight it off. The most common way for immune systems to get enough exposure to these illnesses in order to be able to fight them off when they encounter them is through vaccines.

A vaccine is a combination of the inactive strain of the illness and other things to help deliver that strain properly. When the inactive strain of the illness is properly introduced into your system, the antibodies and the immune system has a chance to identify the illness completely and break it down without too much issue in most cases. Once it's been able to fight off that illness once, the nearest time it encounters it in the active form, the immune system is equipped to handle it much more readily than it would otherwise be. This is why vaccinations are so important in society; to prevent earlier eliminated illnesses from becoming a threat to public health once again.

3. INCUBATION PERIOD

Noun. The period of time between one's exposure to an illness or infection and the development or appearance of symptoms.

This is the period of time it takes from the moment of initial exposure for symptoms to develop. It's typically given in a range, as many illnesses can vary in the time they take to fully develop depending on many factors like your immune system health, where you are, the severity of the exposure, and some other factors.

When an illness enters the body, the warm temperatures and all the things inside the body can help to grow and feed the illness before it has the chance to be treated. In this time, it can multiply, it can change, it can get stronger, and it can even mutate. This is why it's so important that treatment be sought out as quickly as possible for illnesses that can't go away or be treated without medical care.

For COVID-19, the average incubation period is from two day to two weeks. You can still experience the onset of symptoms outside that range, but within that range is when it's most likely. If you notice that you spent some time with someone who was recently in a place that had a lot of patients with COVID-19 (even if they showed no symptoms) and a day proximate, you feel like you're coming down with something, seek medical attention immediately.

Some people are "carriers," which means they can give people the illness, but it hasn't taken hold in their system yet. There are no symptoms to identify carriers, so they're walking around spreading the illness with no idea that they're even doing it. This is why it's incredibly important to make sure that you are keeping yourself clean and healthy and that you're not touching things in a public space, then touching your face. For more information on how best to prevent the spread of illness, see Episode Four.

4. OUTBREAK

Noun. The occurrence of more cases than would normally

be accepted in a particular area at that time.

Outbreak is the phrase that is typically used to call attention to a rash of illnesses without putting the label of "epidemic" on an illness. It still calls attention to the situation at hand, letting the public know that something could be wrong, but doesn't indicate that thousands of people are affected by the illness at one time.

5. PANDEMIC

Noun. An illness or disease that has become prevalent or widely affecting parts of an entire country, or the whole world.

Now, certain illnesses can be experienced all over the world. You are just as likely to get the flu in Canada as you are to get it in Poland, depending on the conditions and the medical care available. For an illness to be considered pandemic, all the cases that span across the country or across continents must be active simultaneously.

Some pandemics can be more severe than others, as some illnesses that have become pandemic are largely treatable, and the range of cases that constitutes a pandemic can be quite varied. Just make sure that, if you get wind that something is a pandemic, you look at the numbers before becoming too alarmed.

In addition to the raw numbers of how many cases, how many deaths, and how many recoveries, you look at the time it took for those numbers to rise. If it leaped up by 300 cases in a single day recently, you could say that there is cause for worry. However, if you found that the number of cases occurring is on the downswing (i.e. only ten cases in one day when earlier days were in the hundreds), things are quickly being reeled back in.

6. QUARANTINE

Noun. This state or period of being isolated or sequestered from the general population to allow an illness to take its course without spreading to others.

Verb. To place someone in such a state of isolation for such purposes.

You may have heard that many people are being quarantined, particularly in areas where there is a large outbreak. This is typically done to keep the illness from spreading to too many people in too short a time. You will generally see quarantines lasting for about two weeks.

By mitigating the spread of an illness, you can keep more people from getting sick and from missing out on the medical care they need in order to recover safely and quickly.

If you are placed in a quarantine, you will need to make provisions for yourself to keep yourself safely in your home for the duration of your quarantine. Some people are permitted to stay in their homes, while others are kept in a medical facility to ensure that if any care is needed during this time, access is fast and simple.

FINAL CHAPTER: WHAT'S NEXT?

No one can predict where the virus will go from here with 100 percent certainty. But it is known that the coronavirus is picking up speed and is also having an increasingly easier time infecting new people. This is a potentially good news/bad news situation.

The bad news is that many more people will become ill, and it's possible that approximately 2-3 percent of them will die.

The good news is that the virus is already mutating to ensure its survival. And in order to survive, it must weaken itself enough to be spread more widely. In other words, killing patients isn't the goal for a virus like this. Instead, mass replication is the goal, and this requires a weaker virus.

This doesn't mean that you shouldn't take the 2019 Wuhan Novel Coronavirus/COVID-19 seriously. As of March 2, 2020, it's a very serious disease that can cause great harm and has been found on six continents and more than 70 nations. It's expected to continue spreading across the U.S. and many other countries. The best thing to do is stay informed and put the earlier listed health tips into action. With any luck, you won't end up needing these tips, but all of them can still help make you healthier in the long run.

Thank you for reading this guide on coronavirus. This is the 5th book I've written since 2016.

It usually takes me years to write a book, also because I am a full-time dad beside being a doctor. The main reason, however, is that I decided to challenge myself even more this time.

My goal for this guide was to put complex concepts in the simplest and quickest way possible, so as to make it readable and readily accessible for everyone.

I accurately selected what I believe are the most useful and effective pieces of advice for you.

I don't like to call myself an author, yet I have to admit that I learned a lot while writing books over the past few years. In fact, what I got from those past publications was validation from readers who enjoyed my work and encouraged me to keep writing.

I always value the opinion of readers and take into account criticism as well.

I do believe that reviews are a great way to give someone credit for the work done, and I love reading them all the time.

Other readers will do the same before purchasing my books; that's why I give special importance to reviews and I feel bad when getting a bad one.

Anyway, I hope you keep in mind that I am a self-published author without the huge possibilities that publishing houses have (such as proofreading, special formatting and so on...).

I hope I accomplished at least the main goal I had in my mind - which was to provide you with useful information about Covid-19, based on medical studies as well as my own 30+ years experience.

Special thanks go to my family, in particular to my beloved wife and my two children, who supported me while writing this book; they read it before than anyone else. I got great feedback from them and I am elated about that, even though I think theirs are a little bit biased. After all, they saw me when at nights, often after exhausting workdays at the hospital, I locked myself up in the study room, writing and organizing this guide in the best possible way.

I hope you will keep that in mind too and consider using some seconds of your precious time to leave a nice review on this book.

I will be *grateful* for each one of you.

P.S. I'm a veteran doctor, I am a dad, but above all... I **am a human being**. An immaculate work is far from possible, especially when you are alone and try to put together as much information as you can. So, please, if you wish to report any typos or inaccuracies you encountered in this guide, please consider emailing me at **doctorelliotcarson@gmail.com**. I will do my best to answer you and make the requested adjustments.

CPSIA information can be obtained
at www.ICGtesting.com
Printed in the USA
LVHW052018071120
671045LV00005B/406

9 781801 157001